eat
5

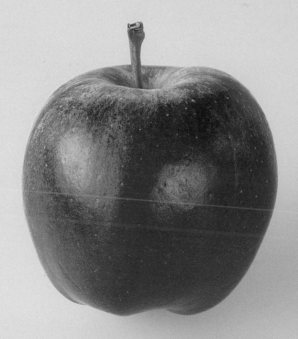

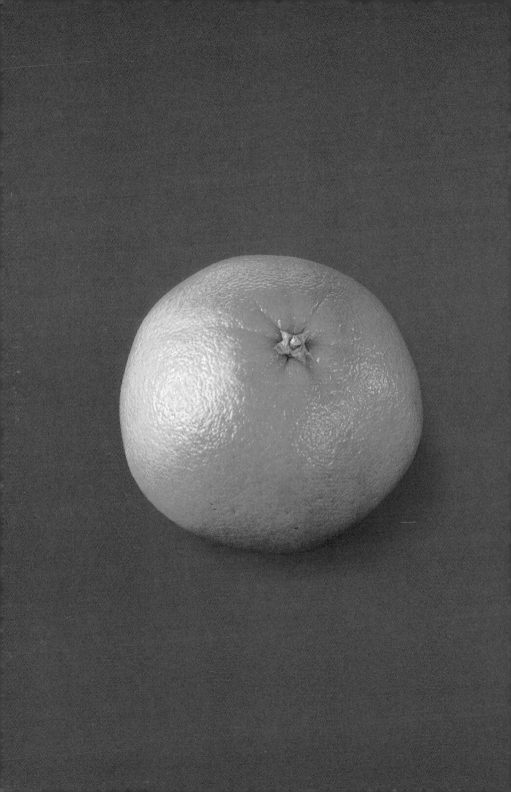

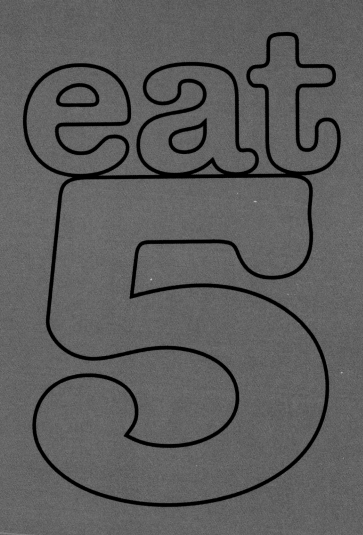

hamlyn

eat 5

CHOOSE THE HEALTHY WAY
WITH 5 FRUIT & VEG A DAY!

Helen Foster

First published in Great Britain in 2002 by
Hamlyn, a division of Octopus Publishing Group Ltd
2–4 Heron Quays, London E14 4JP

ISBN 0 600 60569 8

A CIP catalogue record for this book is available from the British Library

Printed and bound in China

10 9 8 7 6 5 4 3 2

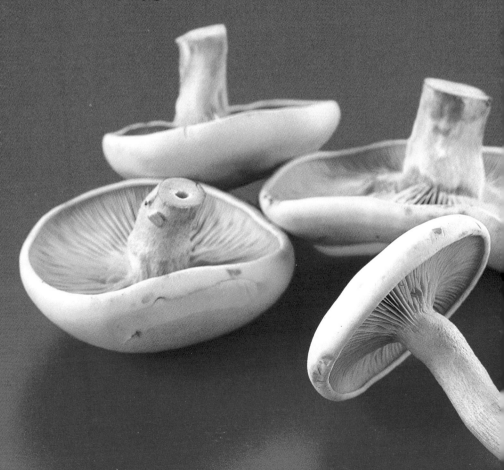

Contents

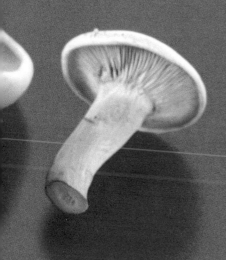

Introduction

Imagine there was a magic pill which, if used regularly, offered protection against cancer and heart disease, helped keep your skin and eyes bright and your weight down, and could be the reason you live longer than those around you. You'd be signing up for a prescription, wouldn't you? The truth is, that although that pill doesn't exist, the benefits do ... and all it takes to get them is a daily dose of fruit and vegetables in your diet.

Remember those brussels sprouts your mother used to force down you when you were a child? Well, doctors now believe they could be one of the most potent preventers of cancers on the planet today. And the apple that supposedly kept the doctor away? It now it seems it did, with doctors at England's Nottingham University finding just 1 apple a day helps strengthen lung function, reducing the risk of respiratory problems like asthma. If you add that to research at the University of Buffalo, USA, which found that people with the strongest lung function were also those who lived the longest, you're looking at some major health benefits. In fact, scientists all over the world are now discovering that **_it's never been truer that we are what we eat_** – and that if what you eat is a diet high in fresh fruit and vegetables what you'll be is healthier, more energized and potentially on your way to a longer life. The best news about all of this is that it doesn't take bucketsful of fruit or vegetables to have this effect. According to the World Health Organization, to get the protective benefits of fruit and vegetables means eating just 5 portions of them every day.

However, the problem is that most of us don't eat that magic 5 figure. Research from the British Food Standards Agency has shown that in the UK only 17 per cent of the population reach 5 portions, with 49 per cent managing just 1 or 2. In the USA, the Department of Agriculture has found that 51 per cent of the population don't eat the recommended 3 portions of vegetables, and 71 per cent don't get the desired 2 portions of fruit. In fact, the only countries where a significant number of the population reach recommended intake levels are the Mediterranean countries like Spain and Greece. Yet, while the figures vary, the reasons for why we don't eat the necessary 5 portions of fruit and vegetables don't.

All around the world people believe the same 3 things:

1. That fruit and vegetables are boring and taste dull;

2. That, to do you any good, you've got to eat raw fruit and vegetables, which isn't always possible in a busy modern world;

3. That 5 portions of fruit and vegetables is a huge amount that can't be integrated into a normal diet.

In fact, none of those things is true; and this is where this book is about to change your life. It will teach you just how easy it is to integrate fruit and vegetables into your world – in other words, how to harness all those powers promised from that magic pill in your life now without any hassle. You're not going to have to become a slave to a steamer, or shop only in organic fruit markets for the foods you'll eat that day. You'll be able to eat desserts, kids' favourites like frozen peas and baked beans, and even smoothies and juices, and know that they're doing you good. In fact, I'm going to show you the simplest, easiest way to transform your health.

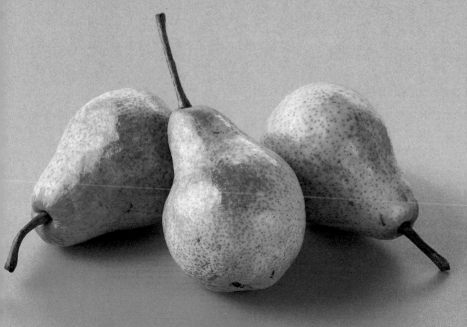

Are you getting enough?

Many of us don't realize exactly what a portion of fruit and vegetables is – and, even if you do have a good idea, other factors may come into play that mean you're not quite getting all the goodness you need from your fruit and vegetables. The first step in your new healthy life is therefore finding out how you do. To do that you need to try the quiz below. It's easy; just check which answer sounds right for you, and then turn to the answers on pages 10–11.

1. **Which of these is a portion?**

a) a medium jacket potato

b) 1 tablespoon of dried apricots

c) 1 tablespoon of frozen peas

d) half an orange

2. **Some surprising things count as portions. Which of these would you class as a fruit or vegetable?**

a) a strawberry yogurt

b) a tablespoon of tomato ketchup

c) a can of baked beans

d) a cupful of nuts

3. **How many of your daily portions can come from juices?**

a) none

b) 1

c) 2

d) 3

4. **How many portions of brussels sprouts, broccoli, cabbage, kale or cauliflower do you eat in a week?**

a) none

b) 1

c) 2

d) 3

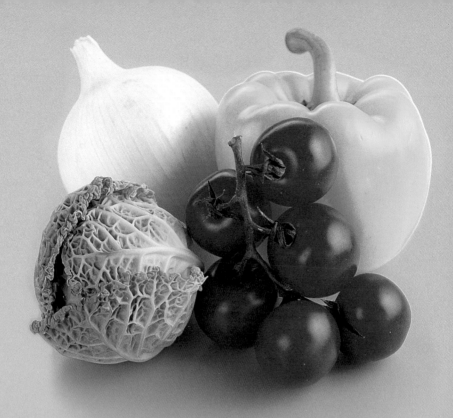

5. Which of the following colours of fruit and vegetables did you eat yesterday?

a) green

b) red

c) yellow

d) white

6. What colour are your eyes?

a) blue or green

b) brown

7. Which of these activities do you do regularly?

a) smoke

b) drink alcohol

c) exercise

Your results

1. The correct answer is **(b)**, and if you're counting any of the others as a portion you may not be getting enough. This may surprise you, as the most common misconception regarding fruit and vegetables is that potatoes count as a vegetable. They don't – they are classed as a starchy food. The other 2 answers are wrong because the portion sizes aren't big enough.

2. The correct answer is **(c)** – baked beans are classed as a vegetable. The first 2 answers don't count as they don't contain enough fruit or vegetable to count as a portion. Nuts don't count as a fruit or a vegetable, although they can be part of a healthy diet.

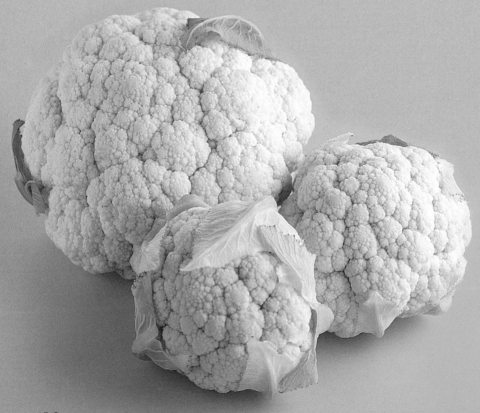

3. No matter how much juice you drink, only answer **(b)** is actually right here. While juices are a great way to get a portion of fruit or vegetables a day, that's all they can be – just 1 portion, as they don't contain enough fibre to truly do your health good. If you've been counting more glasses of juice a day as portions, you could be missing out on some vital benefits. It doesn't mean you can't drink your nutrients, but switch a couple of portions from juices to smoothies (see pages 52–54). As these contain the whole fruit, they count as more than 1 portion.

4. All these vegetables are so-called cruciferous types, of which doctors say you should eat 3 portions a week. This means you score top points if you marked answer **(d)**, but if you picked any of the others you could be lacking in plant protection, no matter how many other fruit and vegetables you eat.

5. The answer that means you're doing OK nutritionally should be all of them – you should have ticked **(a)**, **(b)**, **(c)** and **(d)**. Getting a good variety of colours of fruit and vegetables is the best way to boost your intake of all the beneficial nutrients they contain.

6. This might sound like a strange question, but if your answer was **(a)** you actually need more of some nutrients than your brown-eyed cousins if you want to protect your eyesight.

7. Like having blue or green eyes, all of these activities actually increase your need for certain nutrients.

So, how did you do? The chances are that you slipped up somewhere. You're only human, after all; but it doesn't mean you can't change your habits – and all the advice you need to help you do it is contained in this book.

20 reasons to eat 5

1. The World Health Organization has found that around 85 per cent of adult cancers are avoidable and, of these, about half are related to nutrition deficiencies in the western diet – many of which can be rectified by including those 5 portions of fruit and vegetables.

2. In the USA, heart disease accounts for more than 1 million deaths annually. In Britain, 1 person dies every 3 minutes from coronary heart disease, but new research from Cambridge University has found that eating just 1 apple a day cuts your risk of premature death from heart disease by 20 per cent. Add 1 orange and 1 banana and that increases to 50 per cent.

3. Minor infections such as colds and flu are also less likely. Fruit and vegetables (particularly kiwi fruit, raspberries, blueberries, red peppers and citrus fruit) are the best ways to get high levels of vitamin C in your diet, and research shows that people with high intakes of vitamin C have 34 per cent fewer sick days than others.

4. A 1998 study showed that a high-fibre diet will protect against breast cancer and prostate cancer. There is fibre in nearly all vegetables and in most fruit. Cabbages, peas, beans, berries and dried fruit are all particularly rich sources.

5. Age-related memory loss is one of the most distressing elements of old age, but a 1999 study published in the *Journal of Neuroscience* found that a diet containing the equivalent of half a cup of blueberries a day can actually cause the growth of new brain cells, which may prevent memory deterioration.

6. Most of us think that only dairy products can help build bones, but in fact dark green leafy vegetables such as broccoli and kale can also provide calcium. Onions also help build bones by stopping the process that causes bones to weaken. Studies from the University of Bern in Switzerland found just 1 g of onion a day is enough to strengthen your skeleton.

7. 5 portions a week of red fruit and vegetables (such as tomatoes and watermelon) can reduce the risk of lung cancer by a quarter.

8. Skin cancer caused by ultraviolet (UV) damage is increasing across the world. In Queensland, Australia, 4 out of every 5 people suffer some form of skin cancer, and even in the UK rates for the most dangerous form of skin cancer, melanoma, have at least doubled since 1971. However, research at the University of Arizona has shown that a diet of 5–10 portions of red, yellow or orange fruit and vegetables can reduce skin cancer risk by forming a UV-protection layer under the skin.

9. According to the world's largest study on successful weight loss, focusing on a diet high in fruit and vegetables is a vital factor in losing weight and keeping it off. This is not surprising when you think that a 2–3 tablespoon portion of most fruit or vegetables contains just 50 calories – the same as half a chocolate biscuit or 5 potato crisps.

10. A high intake of fruit and vegetables has been shown to lower the risk of stomach cancer. A Swedish research study on sets of twins found that a twin eating a high intake of fruit and vegetables had 5.5 times less risk of stomach cancer than their brother or sister who did not eat a high intake of fruit and vegetables.

11. Fruit and vegetables can help a number of 'female troubles'. Research from Rutgers University in the USA found that compounds in cranberries and blueberries actually stop bacteria sticking to the inside of the urinary tract, therefore preventing infections like cystitis from taking hold. A glass of cranberry juice or a fistful of blueberries a day is enough to cut frequency of attacks by 58 per cent. Italian research has also found that women eating a high intake of green vegetables had half the normal chance of developing fibroids than those eating fewer vegetables.

12. Fruit and vegetables fight wrinkles. According to research at Monash University in Australia, people with diets high in fresh produce had smoother and less lined skin than those eating diets high in red meat and sugar.

13. Eating 2½ carrots a day has been shown to lower cholesterol by 11 per cent in just 3 weeks in Scottish studies. High cholesterol is one of the major risk factors for heart disease.

14. A 12-year study in the USA showed a significant reduction in strokes among people who consumed a high level of potassium. Fresh fruit and vegetables – particularly bananas, grapes, leeks and cabbages – all provide plenty of potassium.

15. Fruit doesn't even need to be whole to have beneficial effects. According to a study by Harvard University, USA, just 1 glass of orange or grapefruit juice each day may reduce the risk of stroke by a quarter.

16. On average, we need 8 glasses of water a day to keep us functioning on full power – if that hydration level drops by just 2 per cent so do our energy, mental speed and muscle power. Eating 5 portions of fruit and vegetables a day provides the equivalent fluid of 3 glasses of water – more if you choose water-heavy foods like melon, cucumber, celery or lettuce.

17. People who eat 3 portions of broccoli a week reduce the risk of colon cancer by half compared to those who don't eat broccoli. Analysis of studies made at the American National Cancer Institute in 1987 showed that the more cruciferous vegetables (broccoli, cauliflowers, turnips, brussels sprouts, kale, cabbages) that you eat, the lower your chances of developing cancer of the colon.

18. Cataracts are the major cause of blindness in the world – affecting 15–20 million people – and, according to research at Tufts University in Boston, USA, eating less than 1½ portions of fruit and vegetables a day increases your risk of developing them by 600 per cent. Of all the eye-friendly vegetables, spinach seems to score the highest – not only does it help cataracts, but it's also a leading preventative of age-related macular degeneration, the commonest cause of blindness in people over 55.

19. The UK has the highest rate of asthma in the world, with 23 per cent of children aged 6–7 now suffering. In the USA, 15 million people suffer. Even New Zealand, a country renowned for its clean air, sees 1 in 6 suffering. However, UK research published in 2001 found that eating tomatoes every other day – or 1 apple every day – decreased the affects of asthma.

20. One of the most damaging elements of modern life is stress, yet studies show that people eating diets high in fruit and vegetables that contain vitamin B6 (such as bananas and avocados) found it easier to handle stress than those who did not. On average, we need 2 mg of B6 daily – the average banana contains 0.7 mg, an avocado 1.76 mg.

Why 5 portions?

Now you can see why fruit and vegetables can help improve your health, you're probably asking why 5 portions a day is the magic number, when studies are showing that just 1 fruit or 1 portion of vegetables can help combat conditions like heart disease and asthma. Well, quite simply, **while 1 fruit is good, 4 or 5 are even better.** In addition, 5 portions of fruit and vegetables constitute around 400 g (14 oz) of produce – this is the amount that the World Health Organization has estimated also provides us with the 20–30 g (around 1 oz) of fibre we should eat in a day, plus at least the minimum doses of all the vital vitamins and minerals we need to stay healthy.

What doesn't count?

Potatoes: These are classed as a starchy food, not a vegetable. You should aim for 10 portions of starchy foods a day, however, so don't skip them in your diet.

Nuts and seeds: Again, these are healthy foods, but they aren't classed as fruit or vegetables.

Wine: It may be made of grapes, and it may have very high levels of flavonoids, but it doesn't count as a portion.

Tea: This is controversial, as some US experts do class 3 cups of green tea as a portion, and it's been shown to have amazing health benefits. For an all-round health boost, however, it doesn't qualify.

Fruit drinks, squashes and fruit-flavoured waters: These don't include enough real fruit to count.

Jam, marmalade and fruit yogurts: Again, none contains enough fruit to count.

Ketchup: While real tomato sauces and pastes can count as part of your portions, ketchup can't – nor can the tomato sauce in baked beans or tinned spaghetti.

However, the more we learn about fruit and vegetables the more experts are refining those results. Generally, vegetables seem to be showing slightly more health benefits than fruit. Teams from top health centres, like Mount Sinai School of Medicine in New York, are therefore saying that the 5 portions should ideally be split into 3 of vegetables and 2 of fruit. Also, within these, you should aim to have: 1 high beta-carotene food a day (this means mainly red, yellow or orange fruit and vegetables); 1 vitamin C rich food a day (try kiwi fruit, blueberries, raspberries, citrus fruit, red peppers or sweet potatoes), and at least 3 portions from the cruciferous family (such as cauliflowers, cabbages, spinach, broccoli, radishes, turnips, swedes and brussels sprouts) a week. As well as that, you need to ensure a good variety of other fruit and vegetables – the more types you eat, and **the more colours you mix into your diet each day, the higher the variety of phytonutrients (beneficial plant chemicals) you'll get.**

There is no problem with eating more than 5 portions, should you wish. Before you start totting things up, however, you need to know exactly how big a portion is. Studies from the British Dietetic Association have recently shown that many of us are a bit confused about how much we need to eat. The portion sizes on pages 18–21 have been calculated from information compiled by the British Dietetic Association, the American Dietetic Association and health advocacy group The Center for Science in the Public Interest in Washington DC. As recommended portion sizes do vary slightly from group to group, where discrepancies occurred the highest figure has been used.

What's a portion?

Large fruit	Cantaloupe melons, grapefruits, mangos, papayas, pineapples, watermelons
Medium fruit	Apples, avocados, bananas, oranges, peaches, pears
Small fruit	Apricots, clementines, figs, kiwi fruit, passion fruit, plums, satsumas, tomatoes
Berry-type fruit	Blackberries, blackcurrants, blueberries, cherries, cranberries, gooseberries, grapes, raspberries, strawberries
Stewed, tinned and mixed fruit	Apples, apricots, fruit cocktail, fresh fruit salad, peaches, pears, pineapples
Dried fruit	Apricots, bananas, cranberries, dates, figs, papaya, pineapple, raisins, sultanas
Fruit juice	All actual fruit juices, including tomato, freshly squeezed or processed, not fruit drinks

A 'large slice' is roughly an 8th of a very large fruit like watermelon, and half of smaller ones like papaya; a 'cup' is the size of an average coffee mug; and a 'medium glass' holds 150 ml

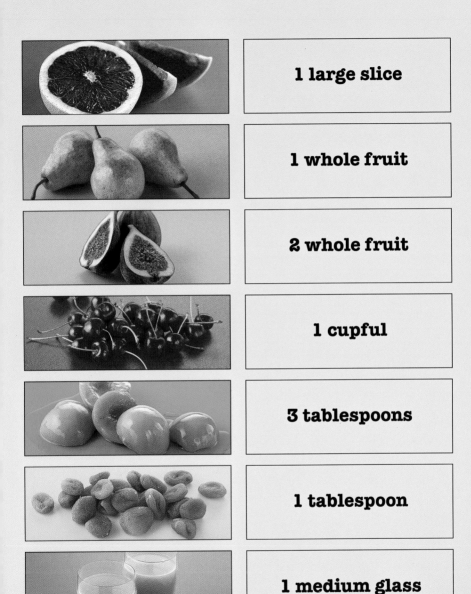

1 large slice

1 whole fruit

2 whole fruit

1 cupful

3 tablespoons

1 tablespoon

1 medium glass

(5 fl oz) of liquid. Fruit juice may only be counted as 1 portion per day, as it doesn't contain as much fibre as whole fruit.

Mixed salad vegetables	Celery, cucumber, iceberg and other pale lettuces
Cruciferous vegetables	Broccoli, brussels sprouts, cabbage, cauliflower, radishes, turnips, swedes
Dark green leafy vegetables	Chard dark green winter cabbage, kale, pak choi, rocket, romaine lettuce, spinach
Other vegetables	Aubergines, carrots, green beans, mushrooms, onions, peas, peppers, squashes
Sprouting beans	Alfalfa, beansprouts, broccoli sprouts
Beans and pulses	Baked beans, black beans, chickpeas, kidney beans, lentils, soya beans
Vegetable juice	Beetroot, carrot, wheatgrass

A 'cup' is the size of an average coffee mug, and a 'medium glass' holds 150 ml (5 fl oz) of liquid. Beans and pulses may only be counted as one portion per day; this also applies to vegetable juice.

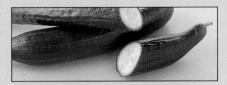 1 dessert bowlful

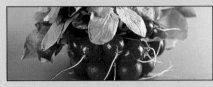 2 tablespoonfuls

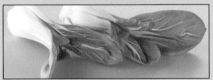 2 tablespoonfuls

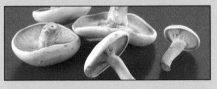 2 tablespoonfuls

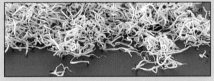 Half a cupful

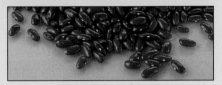 Half a cupful

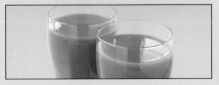 1 medium glass

What's in fruit and vegetables?

Each fruit or vegetable contains 'active ingredients' that make it what it is, and scientists are finding that these ingredients (called phytochemicals or phytonutrients) react with our bodies to prevent disease. Nobody knows how many of these vital substances exist in plants, but here are some of the most important discovered so far.

Anti-oxidant vitamins

The main causes of damage and ageing in our bodies are molecules called free radicals, which destroy cells and tissues. This destruction is believed to be responsible for most cancers, for the furring of the arteries that leads to heart attacks, for the degeneration of the skin that causes wrinkles – and a whole host of other nasty things. If left unchecked, they are lethal; however, when a free radical meets an anti-oxidant the 2 bind and the free radical's destructive power is neutralized. Many vitamins and minerals are anti-oxidants, but those most commonly found in fruit and vegetables are primarily vitamin C and beta-carotene (a carotenoid – see below – which turns into vitamin A). Good sources of vitamin C are kiwi fruit and citrus fruits, while pumpkins, sweet potatoes and carrots supply high levels of beta-carotene.

Carotenoids

Carotenoids (like lycopene, beta-carotene and lutein) are the substances in plants that give them their red, yellow or orange colour. They work mainly by being very powerful anti-oxidants, but they also have other actions in the body. For example, lutein is believed to create an actual UV-filter in the back of the eye, preventing damaging light hitting the retina and reducing the risk of age-related blindness;other carotenoids seem to detect the presence of pre-cancerous cells in the body and send out messages to the cells to prevent them from growing. Not surprisingly, carotenoids are found primarily in red and orange foods (such as peppers, sweet potatoes, oranges and watermelons), but also appear in dark green leafy vegetables like broccoli, spinach and kale.

Flavonoids

When they were first discovered, flavonoids were called vitamin P. However, they were stripped of this name because, for a substance to be a vitamin, it must be proved that if it is missing from the diet negative symptoms occur. This doesn't happen with flavonoids – if you don't eat them you don't get sick – but that doesn't mean they are not essential to health. The more scientists look at flavonoids the more positive effects in the body they find – they are anti-allergens, they are anti-inflammatory, they stimulate the immune system and they impede the growth of cancers. Like carotenoids, there are many types of flavonoid – flavonols found in apples and onions, and anthocyanidins found in berries, for example – but all are vital for our health.

Fibre

Fibre is a catch-all name for the structural parts of fruit and vegetables – things like cellulose and pectin that make up the cells of the plant and give it form. Surprisingly, fibre has no nutritional value to us at all. It doesn't contain vitamins and minerals, and it doesn't contain calories; in fact, we don't even digest some of it. Yet this doesn't mean that it doesn't have a vital health role to play. Fibre's main function is to help us with the excretion of foods – without it, the risk of constipation (and other bowel disorders) is increased. However, scientists are now discovering other potential roles for fibre – it has been shown to lower cholesterol; its ability to fill us up is a major part of successful weight loss; and a high intake has been linked to a lowered risk of many digestive or bowel cancers.

Glucosinolates

Found in cruciferous vegetables like cabbages, cauliflowers and brussels sprouts, these compounds are the body's detoxifiers. They help provide the liver with what it needs to tackle toxins but, more importantly, they can help to ward off cancer-causing agents. They also help to regulate white blood cells and strengthen the immune system to fight against invaders. Glucosinolates come in different forms (the one you may have heard about is called sulforaphane, which is found in brussels sprouts) and each acts in a different part of the body but the more scientists find out about them the more important they seem to be. In fact, some cancer researchers have even gone as far as to say that glucosinolates could be the most vital weapon we have in the fight against cancer.

Other vitamins and minerals

While the anti-oxidant vitamins may hit the headlines, fruit and vegetables contain many other vital vitamins and minerals as well. To be in optimum health, the human body actually needs a delicate balance of 59 vitamins and minerals – and, of these, all can be found to some extent in fruit and vegetables. For example, 1 banana contains 10 per cent of the heart-helping potassium we need in a day, and just 1 cup of spinach provides a fifth of the iron.

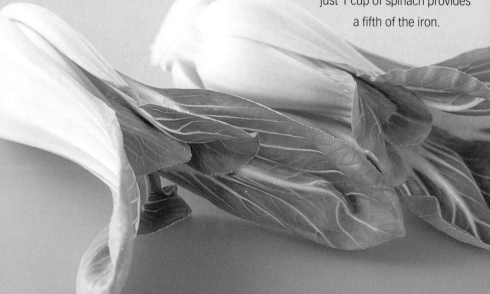

Phytoestrogens

Breast cancer is the second most common female cancer in the world and in many cases the tumour's growth is influenced by the presence of the hormone oestrogen. However, because they have a structure very similar to oestrogen, phytoestrogens can help to prevent this happening. They do this by entering the part of the cell oestrogen would normally infiltrate, and blocking it. Since oestrogen can't enter the cell, it can't stimulate tumour growth. Their presence in the diet is thought to be one reason why almost 6 times fewer women die of breast cancer in Japan than in the UK. Trials are also looking at their effects on prostate cancer in men. You'll find the highest quantities of phytoestrogens in soya bean based products such as endame, and in some soya milks, yogurts and breads containing soya, but they also occur in sprouting beans such as alfalfa.

Sterols

Normally found in the seeds of plants, sterols are actually a form of fat that occurs in small quantities in plant fibres. Chemically, they are very similar to cholesterol, and when they enter the gut they actually compete with cholesterol (from diet and bile) reducing the amount that can be absorbed. In fact, research in the *European Journal of Clinical Nutrition* found that just 1.6 g of plant sterols a day lowered cholesterol on average by 10 per cent. Sterols also act on the immune system, increasing the activity of the main fighting cells (called natural killer cells) which destroy bacteria – and cancer cells – when they are present. In fact, studies in South Africa have used supplements of sterols to actually reverse early-stage cervical cancer. While the best sources of plant sterols are supplemented food products such as mayonnaise and yogurts they are also found in green and yellow vegetables, peanuts and beans such as kidney beans and chickpeas, classed as part of your daily fruit and vegetable intake.

Top 10 fruit

While all fruit contains healthy ingredients, there are some that are better at protecting our health than others.

Apples

A team at Cornell University in New York found that 1 apple provides the same amount of usable vitamin C as 1.5 g taken in supplement form. Apples also score highly in the top 10 of fruit people enjoy eating – which is a big plus, as studies also show the scent of apples can prevent migraine in people that like the fruit. It's thought to trigger pleasure sensations in the body which stop the pain.

Avocados

These contain the highest concentration of the vital anti-oxidant vitamin E of any fruit. They score top for fruit in their content of eye-protecting lutein, and provide 3 times more of a substance called glutathione than any other fruit – glutathione may reduce the risk of oral cancers. Avocados are also rich in monounsaturated fats which can help to lower cholesterol.

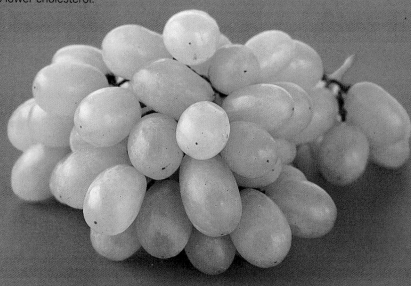

Blueberries

When researchers looked into which fresh fruit had the highest percentage of anti-oxidants, they found it was blueberries. Just half a cup doubles the amount of anti-oxidants the average person gets in a day. They can help to beat the memory loss and coordination problems that can occur as we age.

Cranberries

Like all berries, these are high in anti-ageing anti-oxidants, and they can help reduce cystitis. New research also shows they can help teeth by stopping the bacteria that cause plaque from sticking to the teeth.

Grapes

As well as containing fibre and anti-oxidants in their skin, grapes contain a substance called resveratrol. This protects grapes from fungal disease, but it helps us by reducing the risk of heart disease. Grape juice may even be more protective than whole fruit as it contains the seeds that have high levels of heart-healthy flavonoids.

Kiwi fruit

In 1997, the *Journal of the American College of Nutrition* published a list of the most nutritionally dense fruit, and discovered that – despite its size – 1 kiwi fruit provides you with the recommended amount of vitamin C you need in a day. It's also full of eye-aiding lutein, constipation-, cholesterol- and cancer-fighting fibre, the minerals copper, potassium and magnesium, and even a dose of vitamin E.

Prunes

These dried plums are the ultimate anti-oxidant foods, providing twice as many anti-oxidants as blueberries, the fresh fruit with the highest level of anti-oxidants. The reputation of prunes to beat constipation, which can cause many digestive ailments including some cancers, is also well deserved. As well as fibre, prunes contain tartaric acid (a natural laxative) and dihydrophenyl isatin which triggers the intestine to contract.

Raspberries

Take note of the name ellagic acid, because over 125 studies have shown that this phytonutrient may play a role in defeating and preventing cancer – particularly of the breast or cervix. The little seeds on the sides of your raspberries are the highest source of ellagic acid. Raspberries are also high in vitamin C and provide fibre. In fact, 1 cup contains more fibre than the same weight of bran flakes.

Strawberries

Like raspberries, strawberries are high in ellagic acid. They're also high in vitamin C and fibre. Just 8 berries will provide you with a fifth of the folic acid a non-pregnant person needs in a day. If you're exposed to passive smoking, strawberries could help. Researchers at Indiana and Ohio Universities found they reduce the effects of benzopyrene, a carcinogen in tobacco smoke.

Watermelon

Lycopene is a vital anti-cancer agent. While watermelon contains less per gram than tomatoes, the fact that you eat larger portions means, on average, you take in almost 4 times as much lycopene per portion. Also, watermelon provides the equivalent of a glass of water a slice, helping to prevent both dehydration and fluid retention.

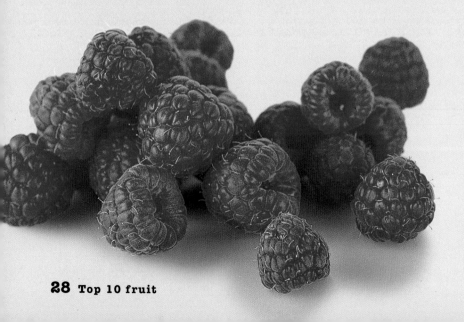

Top 10 vegetables

Bell peppers

These help fight cancer, the effects of ageing, and heart disease. A green pepper provides twice as much vitamin C as a citrus fruit, and a red pepper provides 3 times as much. They are also high in beta-carotene again, red peppers provide 9 times as much as a green pepper. Red peppers also contain lycopene.

Broccoli

When broccoli enters your body, it switches on the production of an enzyme called mammalian detoxifying enzyme – it's a long name for something that fights cancer-causing chemicals in the body and inhibits tumour growth. Broccoli is also high in calcium, with a portion providing 10 per cent of the recommended daily intake. It is a rich source of folate, vitamin C and the essential mineral selenium.

Brussels sprouts

Like broccoli, sprouts contain ingredients important for detoxifying the body, and they also have high anti-oxidant abilities. Studies from Harvard School of Public Health showed that brussels sprouts were among the top 4 vegetables that lowered stroke risk.

Carrots

Yes, they do help you see in the dark by feeding the light-sensitive area of the eye the vitamin A it needs. Add to this the fact that men who eat carrots have a lower risk of lung cancer than other men, and their cholesterol-lowering properties, and you've got a very beneficial food. Just 1 tip: remove their leafy tops as soon as you buy/pick them, since leaving them on actually reduces nutrient levels.

Garlic

Regular consumption of garlic can knock 13 years off the age of your heart. So say German researchers who have found that garlic helps prevent the stiffening of the arteries that contributes to heart disease. Garlic is also an immune booster and a blood thinner, and may even make you feel happy. Studies at the Smell and Taste Treatment Center in Chicago found that families eating with the scent of garlic bread in the house were nicer to each other than other families.

Onions

In ancient Egypt it was said that onions could cure 28 different diseases, and modern science seems to be proving this right. The most important ingredient in onions is a flavonoid called quercetin which helps strengthen everything from lungs to bones, and is the ingredient in wine that makes it protect your heart. Red onions have higher levels of nutrients than white ones.

Soya beans

A half-cup portion of soya beans contains a third of the phytoestrogens that women need in a day to help prevent breast cancer. They can also reduce menopausal symptoms such as hot flushes. It's not just women who may benefit, though: studies are also suggesting that soya-based products can help fight prostate cancer.

Spinach

Packed with fibre, spinach is also the best eye-protecting food, containing at least 5 times more sight-saving lutein than other foods. It also has energy-giving iron and lots of folic acid, a nutrient proven to reduce the risk of birth defects. Finally, spinach is rich in vitamin K, and studies from Harvard Medical School show that elderly women with the highest intake of vitamin K had a 43 per cent lower risk of hip fracture.

Sweet potatoes

When The Center for Science in the Public Interest of Washington, DC decided to rate vegetables by adding up their content of fibre and 6 vital nutrients (vitamins A and C, folate, iron, copper and calcium), sweet potatoes came out on top. It is easy to see why when you realize they contain as much vitamin A as 23 cups of broccoli, are a very low fat source of vitamin E and contain more fibre than oatmeal cereal.

Tomatoes

Technically, a tomato is a fruit, but most of us regard them as vegetables. Tomatoes are the best source of the vital anti-oxidant lycopene, which has been shown to protect against lung, prostate and cervical cancers. Just 1 tomato-based product a day can cut your risk of lung cancer by 25 per cent.

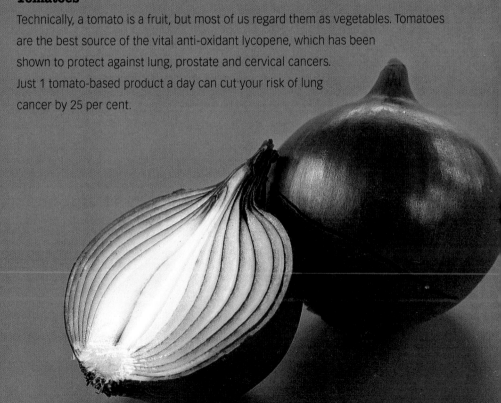

Fresh, frozen or tinned?

Another common misconception about fruit and vegetables is that that frozen or canned varieties just don't measure up to fresh with regard to nutritional value. That's not true – in fact, in some cases **nutrients can actually be greater in frozen or canned foods than in the fresh versions.**

The problem is that, as soon as a fruit or vegetable is picked, the nutrients within it start to deteriorate. If you eat foods within 2 days of being picked, this isn't so much of a problem; but, as most foods take 3–7 days to reach the supermarket, by the time they reach your table some vitamins (particularly those susceptible to damage from light and heat, such as vitamin C or folate) can be reduced by as much as 70 per cent. This doesn't happen with frozen or canned foods. They're processed within hours of being picked, reducing nutrient destruction. In fact, a study from the University of Illinois found that frozen green beans contained twice as much vitamin C as fresh beans sold 7 days after picking. Other foods also thrive on being frozen. While peas lose 33 per cent of their vitamin C during freezing, 50 per cent is lost by being transported or stored for 7 days after picking.

The florets of broccoli contain higher levels of beta-carotene than the stalks. Most frozen-food manufacturers remove the stalks so, weight for weight, frozen broccoli contains 35 per cent more beta-carotene than fresh – although it does contain less calcium. To help frozen peaches retain their colour, manufacturers add vitamin C to them, meaning they contain slightly higher levels than fresh ones.

It's not just frozen foods that score highly nutritionally. Canned ones do too, for, **as well as preserving nutrients, the canning process can also help produce them.** When foods are canned, they are treated with a high-intensity heat, and in some foods this releases nutrients, making them easier for us to use. This is the case with lycopene, with canned tomatoes providing 3 times more than fresh, and tomato paste providing 5 times more.

Boost nutrients in fresh foods

Sometimes there's nothing better than the look and smell of fresh fruit and vegetables. Here's how to ensure you're buying the most nutritious forms:

- Buy locally produced goods, as these will have spent less time in transit and therefore experienced less deterioration; or go to farms and orchards and pick your own.

- Only buy products that look healthy, and avoid anything bruised or split – when air gets into fruit or vegetables, anti-oxidants are destroyed.

- Don't buy goods that are displayed outside or in windows; heat and sunlight also destroy nutrients.

- Store all fruit and vegetables chilled, not in vegetable racks or fruit bowls. Chilling reduces vitamin C deterioration in broccoli by around 40 per cent over one week.

This happens with other nutrients too. Because food manufacturers tend to use the brightest pumpkins for canning, and because the process removes water-concentrating nutrients, canned pumpkin contains 20 times more beta-carotene than fresh. The body sometimes finds it hard to use the fibre in fresh beans; however, the canning process softens the fibre, making it more soluble and therefore more useful to the body.

Of course, some brands of frozen or canned foods do come with other drawbacks. Sugar or salt may have been added, neither of which have any health benefits; so, to eat well using canned or frozen foods, always choose those that state they have no added sugar or salt. Also, beware how you handle canned or frozen foods – damaged cans or defrosted then refrozen packs will lead to nutrient destruction. Store both types of food correctly to get the most benefits and there's no reason why they can't join fresh fruit and vegetables as part of your daily 5 portions.

Raw or cooked?

There are 2 reasons why raw vegetables are generally thought of as more nutritious than cooked ones. First, if you cook vegetables badly you destroy nutrients within them. Studies from the US Department of Agriculture have shown that, when boiled in water, green vegetables such as spinach lose 45 per cent of their vitamin C, 35 per cent of their folate and at least 5 per cent of every other nutrient.

The second reason is slightly more complex, and involves the 'theory of living foods'. In this theory it's believed that, when raw, food is alive and contains high levels of enzymes that our bodies need to digest that food correctly. If you cook food, these enzymes die, and therefore when the food is eaten the body has to make its own enzymes to use in digestion. This prevents it doing other more important things, such as healing diseases or making energy, so it functions less efficiently. Most dietitians don't believe this to be true, primarily because the enzymes in food are destroyed by stomach acid before they can actually do any good, and if we weren't meant to digest food ourselves why would we have a system in place that lets us do it?

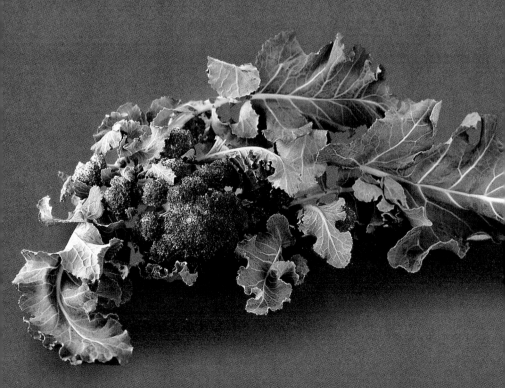

Correct cooking

Vegetables must be cooked properly, however, or the nutrients may be lost. Think about the following.

- Microwaving is the best way to cook fruit and vegetables, as fewer nutrients are destroyed. Steaming and stir-frying are the next most effective methods. Baking can also be good, as nutrients are not leached out in the process.

- Boiling causes most nutrient loss from foods; but, if you do want to boil fresh fruit or vegetables, use as little water as possible and eat them when they are still slightly crunchy.

- Use your cooking water in gravy or sauces (or, if you can stomach it, cool it and then drink it) as it will contain any nutrients lost in the cooking process.

- Keep skins on foods wherever possible, as this prevents some nutrient loss, and cut food items into large chunks rather than little cubes or slices.

- When cooking canned foods, remember they have already been heated and need much less cooking time than fresh or frozen foods.

The final nail in the 'raw is best' coffin, however, comes from recent research presented at a meeting of the American Chemical Society, which showed that cooked carrots actually provided 3 times more beta-carotene than raw ones. The reason for this is that cooking softens the tough cell walls, making it easier for our bodies to absorb the beta-carotene the cells contain. Add this to what we already know about how more lycopene is present in cooked tomatoes, and how the heating during canning helps us use fibre, and it's clear that raw vegetables aren't necessarily better.

Easy ways to eat 5

No matter how busy you are, how late you get up or how much you hate peeling vegetables, it's easily possible to incorporate 5 portions of fruit and vegetables into your day. There are 5 golden rules for success. Even if you just follow these rules and ignore all the tasty recipes and tips that follow, you'll find you can reach that famous 5 target.

The 5 golden rules

1. One at a time

While the idea of sitting down to a salad packed with all 5 portions may excite some of us, for most of us it sounds dull. However, you don't have to get all your portions in one go. The average person eats 3 meals and 2 snacks (or desserts) a day. If, at each of these eating occasions, you make it a rule to get 1 portion of fruit or vegetables, you've hit 5 pretty easily. It can be as simple as a glass of juice at breakfast, a tomato with your sandwich at lunch, some carrot sticks and hummus for a snack, berries and yogurt for dessert and a portion of spinach for dinner (and that's a vegetable you don't even need to cook for it to taste good).

2. Grate, chop, sprinkle

Fruit and vegetables don't even need to show to count. If you add 2 tablespoons of chopped carrots to a prepared soup, mash 2 tablespoons of brussels sprouts into your potato, or sprinkle 1 chopped apple into your muesli in the morning, that's a portion.

3. Think variety

Are you cooking 1 portion of peas? Why not pop a large handful of green or broad beans into the pan too? This will give you double the phytonutrients with no extra fuss.

4. Don't hide the good stuff

If fruit and vegetables are on display, you're more likely to grab them. While it is better to keep produce in the fridge, having a few oranges, plums, bananas or apples in a bowl on the table won't hurt for a day or so – and they'll remind you to grab one as you go past. For best results, put out 4–5 pieces and make it a rule that the bowl must be emptied in 48 hours.

5. Remember convenience counts

If you don't have time to peel and chop fresh vegetables, then eat canned, frozen or pre-prepared varieties instead.

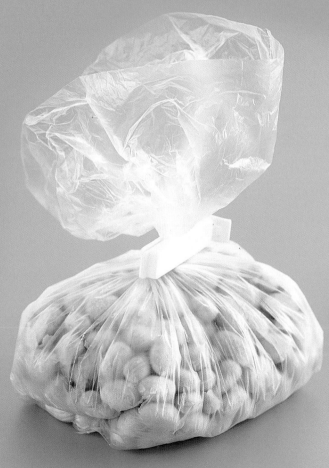

Breakfast

If there's one thing that nutritionists all agree on, it's that breakfast is the most important meal of the day. The main reason is that overnight the body goes into fasting mode, during which it just doesn't work so well. Go to work on an empty stomach and all your systems are impaired. However, eat breakfast and you refuel your blood-sugar supplies and are ready to face the day. In fact, research studies from the University of Wales in Swansea show that ***breakfast-eaters have 22 per cent better memories than those who skip breakfast,*** and trials from Harvard University found that school children who ate breakfast had better grades than those who didn't. When most of us think breakfast, we tend to think carbohydrate foods: cereals, toast, bagels or pastries. Occasionally, we might think protein foods like eggs or bacon but very rarely – other than the odd glass of fruit juice – do we think fruit and vegetables. In fact, studies from the Produce for Better Health Foundation in the USA found only 10 per cent of the breakfast foods we eat are made up of fruit, vegetables, beans or fruit juice. This is not such a smart move – in fact, breakfast is the prime time of day when you should be eating more fruit and vegetables.

One reason for this is the theory of assimilation. According to Swedish research carried out in the 1940s, the body runs in 3 distinct cycles when it focuses on particular tasks, and first thing in the morning there is the assimilation cycle, during which nutrients taken into the body are absorbed in higher concentrations. Another reason is opportunity: it's going to be a lot easier to eat 5 portions by 8pm if you've already downed 2 by 8am. Finally, fruit- and vegetable-based breakfasts may help you keep your weight under control. It's well understood that people who eat breakfast control their weight better than those who skip the meal; but, in a study of overweight children at the Tufts University in Boston, those given a breakfast of a vegetable omelette and a piece of fruit actually ate 81 per cent fewer calories in their next meal than those given cereal and toast, as they just felt fuller for longer. Considering obesity is one of the main risk factors for cancer, heart disease and diabetes, that's not something to be sniffed at.

7 easy ways to eat 5 at breakfast time

1. Drink a glass of fruit juice Maybe orange, grapefruit or apple. All count as 1 portion.

2. Sprinkle a cupful of berries on top of your cereal This makes 1 portion, and its vitamin C content will help boost the absorption of iron from your cereal.

3. Don't top your toast with jam For the same calories as 2 teaspoonfuls of jam, you can mash 1 banana and gain a portion.

4. Smoothies make delicious, nutritious foods that you can eat on the run Combine 1 cupful of blackberries, 1 banana and a cupful of orange juice, and you've got 3 portions in 1 glass.

5. Give the kids beans on toast Why keep their favourite for teatime? A slice of wholemeal bread topped with a small can of beans will keep them fired up until lunch – and provide 1 portion.

6. Try a grilled tomato on toast, or a cupful of mushrooms with scrambled eggs These are 1 portion each.

7. Combine fresh fruit and yogurt Mix 1 chopped apple, 1 tablespoon of chopped apricots and 1 tablespoon of raisins into some low-fat natural yogurt, and you have 3 portions – and a breakfast packed with fibre.

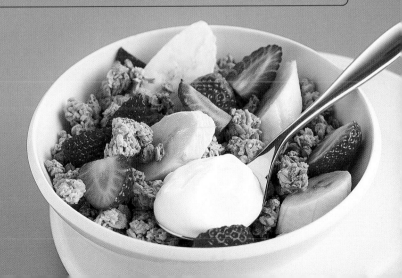

Lunch

Lunch is another meal where many of us miss out on our vital fruit and vegetables. When you're not at home, trying to find fresh, nutritious food can be a chore – and sadly the pickle in your fast-food burger does not add up to a portion. Most of us think it doesn't matter, but in fact not eating your fruit and vegetables at lunchtime could potentially be sapping your performance at work.

6 easy ways to eat 5 at lunchtime

1. **Say yes to spuds** While jacket potatoes themselves don't count as a portion, choosing a vegetable topping, such as bean-based chilli, vegetable curry, ratatouille or even baked beans, is an easy way to chalk up a portion.

2. **Swap pre-packed sandwiches for those made to order in sandwich bars** Also ask them to pop in some extra tomato, dark lettuces like rocket, red onions, alfalfa sprouts and avocado. The average sandwich filled with that lot will provide 1–2 portions.

3. **Bring soup to work in a flask** This will provide a speedy lunch that can be packed with nutrients. You don't even have to make your own – just toss in some extra vegetables like peas, diced carrots, sweetcorn, asparagus or mushrooms when you heat pre-packed varieties. Remember that every 2 tablespoons of vegetables is a portion.

4. **Choose pre-packed salads with less traditional ingredients** Salads based on beans, lentils, chickpeas, carrots or spinach need smaller amounts in order to count as a portion than those based on pale lettuces or cucumber.

5. **Swap that coke for juice** If you didn't use your portion at breakfast, lunchtime juice is the perfect way to get a portion – no matter where you are.

6. **Have dessert** A portion of fruit after your meal will help fill you up (and add nutrients). Choose filling fruit, such as grapes, apples or oranges, for best results.

This is because fresh foods are brain food. Research at the University of Toronto found that the speed and agility of the brain is probably controlled by the amount of blood that reaches it, and that meals high in natural sugars like glucose and fructose boost blood flow. Foods that contain lots of natural sugars include carbohydrate foods such as potatoes and pasta, beans, starchy vegetables like corn, and fruit. Add to this the fact that berries such as blueberries have been shown to boost neuron functioning, and you have good reason to eat more fruit and vegetables at lunchtime.

Yet it isn't the only reason. Fruit and vegetables can also help stop you succumbing to that 3pm sugar fix. There are 2 reasons for this. First, **when some 38 foods were measured by the University of Sydney on their ability to fill you up, oranges, baked beans, bananas, grapes and apples were among the highest scorers.** Second, these foods are among those least likely to cause the sudden falls in blood sugar that tend to cause sugar cravings. These 2 effects combined mean that a lunch based around fruit and vegetables (and ideally a little protein, which maximizes their effects) can stop your sugar cravings. Even if it's stress, not hunger, that sends you on a chocolate run, fruit and vegetables can help. The reason here is that the adrenal glands, which control stress in the body, use vitamin C to help you keep symptoms under control. If you have a low level, they can't work as well and you don't handle stress as well. When you eat more fruit and vegetables, you take in more vitamin C, and the world can seem a better place.

Evening meal

6 easy ways to eat 5 in the evening

1. *If eating ready meals, always serve at least 1 portion of vegetables with them* If time's an issue, choose those that take just 2–3 minutes to cook, such as spinach or asparagus. Spinach is also good as it can be eaten raw (as can broccoli, carrots or salad stuffs); or try canned sweetcorn, peas or carrots, which take much less cooking than fresh or frozen foods.

2. *Add to stews, sauces, soups or casseroles* Whenever you're cooking these, add at least 2 tablespoons of diced fresh or frozen vegetables per person.

3. *Add to pizzas and stir-fries* Pile pizzas with extra vegetables (try mushrooms, peppers, spinach and extra tomato sauce), and bolster up stir-fries with added carrots, peppers and beansprouts.

4. *Fruit needn't be eaten raw to make a great dessert* Stuff a cored apple with 2 tablespoons of raisins and bake at 200°C (400°F) or gas mark 6 for 45 minutes and you've got 2 portions in 1 tasty dish. Or try warming berries and pouring them over vanilla ice cream.

5. *When making mashed potato, add vegetables* Use cabbage, swede, carrots, parsnips, chopped onion or sweetcorn for an extra taste fix –and double the nutrients.

6. *Serve salad before you start* Mixing up fresh starter salads is a great way to boost nutrients – and help curb your appetite for fatty foods. Try high-colour, top-taste combinations like rocket and tomato; spinach and red onion; grated carrot and beetroot; or apple, walnut and celery in natural yogurt.

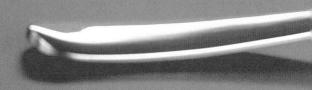

Evening is probably the time most of us will find it easier to fit fruit and vegetables into our diet. We have more time, meals are normally under control, and often they just seem to fit the addition of a couple of portions of green or cruciferous vegetables more than the 'fast' foods we eat at lunchtime.

All of this makes for good nutritional news for our bodies – particularly in terms of family eating habits. A huge American study called the 'Sons of Nurses Health Study' looked at the nutrition of children and found that kids who eat evening meals with their family (rather than at the house of friends, or who snack in front of the TV) are twice as likely to eat all their portions of fruit and vegetables than those who eat alone. These children also have higher levels of vital health-promoting nutrients such as calcium, iron, folate and vitamins C and E.

General nutrition isn't the only benefit brought by using your evening meal to bolster your portions. Let's take the size and shape of your waistline. By focusing your evening meal on fruit and vegetables you could even maximize the weight you are losing on a diet programme. Studies at the US Department of Agriculture found that when people ate larger evening meals (albeit those low in calories) they actually lost a higher percentage of body fat in the weight they lost than those who ate bigger meals in the morning. You can also ***use the fruit and vegetables in your evening meal to ensure you get a good night's sleep.*** Lettuce, for example, contains an opium-like ingredient which helps naturally sedate you, boosting more restful sleep, while bananas encourage your body to produce the calming hormone tryptophan (add a glass of milk to them and this effect is heightened further). For most of us, eating fruit and vegetables in the evening is fairly easy – the average family consumes 75 per cent of their portions then – but to truly follow the Eat 5 programme you need to make those portions count every day.

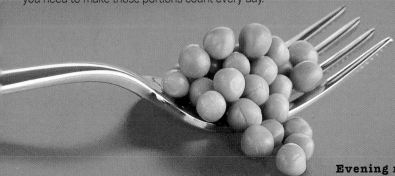

Snacks

The average person snacks twice a day – and most of us do it with a little guilt. Generally, this isn't undeserved, as most of the snacks we choose tend to be laden with fat or sugar. In fact, according to a survey by recruitment agency Office Angels, *57 per cent of people would rather snack on chocolate or crisps than fruit,* and US Government statistics say that Americans eat only 1 vegetable-based snack a month (despite snacking twice a day). This 'fresh snack phobia' isn't such a great idea, since when used correctly snacks can ensure you reach that magic 5 portions, and boost your health.

The thing is, eating 3 medium-sized meals with the odd snack in between was the way our body was designed to eat. Large meals burden the digestive system, often causing bloating and lowered energy while the body struggles to digest them. By eating smaller meals you prevent this, and the body functions more efficiently – particularly if you eat fruit and vegetables, as the body finds these exceptionally easy to digest. A diet that includes fresh food snacks also helps stabilize your blood sugar (see also page 40)

5 supersnacks

1. Chop 2 carrots and eat them dipped in half a cup of salsa to gain 2 portions.

2. A small box of raisins equals 1 portion.

3. Dipping slices of banana in 2 teaspoons of peanut butter makes a fibre-filled taste sensation.

4. Mix a cupful of berries into a low-fat yogurt; if you do this, a fruit yogurt does count as 1 portion.

5. Spear cubes of melon, 8–10 strawberries and a banana on wooden kebab sticks; this provides 3 portions.

Wrap it up

This simple snack can be eaten anywhere; you can even make it at your desk.

2 soft flour tortillas
1 tablespoon hummus
1 cup raw, fresh spinach
half an avocado, sliced
2 tablespoons red and
 yellow peppers, cored,
  deseeded and sliced
1 tomato, diced

1. Spread the tortillas with half the hummus. Now, dividing them equally between the tortillas, lay the spinach leaves over the top – leave about 1 cm (1/2 inch) clear at the bottom of the tortilla.

2. Add the rest of the hummus and sprinkle on the rest of the ingredients, dividing them equally between each tortilla and focusing them in the middle of the wraps.

3. Now fold the bottom of each tortilla up and roll the parcel over to seal it all. Serve with a bean salad, made from half a can of kidney beans mixed with a little oil and vinegar dressing.

and, according to the Medical Research Council's Human Nutrition Research Unit in England, measurements of fatty acids in the blood are also more likely to remain stable when you eat small amounts of food often – which is good news, as peaks and troughs in fatty acid levels have been shown to increase the risk of heart disease.

Finally, by eating fruit and vegetables as snacks you maximize your potential for reaching that magic 5 number of portions, and it really does make a difference to your body. When the nutrition department of Queen Margaret's University College in Edinburgh, Scotland, studied eating patterns of those who snacked on fruit and vegetables, they found they ate less fat and more carbohydrates than other eaters (both of which boost health). Other studies looking into more detailed measurements have found snackers to have higher levels of vitamin C and other nutrients in their system.

To snack properly, base your snacks around fruit and vegetables rather than crisps, chocolate or cakes. Smoothies (see pages 52–54) are also good for filling that gap.

Mega menus

Here are 6 dishes and meals that each provide a whole host of fruit and vegetables. The portions given are for the whole recipe, rather than individual servings.

Mango and avocado salad with smoked chicken

2 ripe avocados
2 tablespoons lemon juice
1 small mango
3 tablespoons olive oil
1 teaspoon wholegrain mustard
1 teaspoon clear honey
2 teaspoons cider vinegar
sea salt and freshly ground black
  pepper
handful of watercress
50 g (2 oz) cooked beetroot,
  finely sliced
175 g (6 oz) smoked chicken,
  thinly sliced

1. Halve, stone and peel the avocados. Either slice or dice the avocado flesh and place in a shallow bowl with the lemon juice. Stir to combine.

2. Cut through the mango either side of the central stone, peel away the skin and slice the flesh.

3. Mix the olive oil with the wholegrain mustard, honey, vinegar, salt and pepper, and mix well. Remove the avocado from the lemon juice and mix the juice into the dressing.

4. Arrange the watercress and beetroot on 4 plates or in a salad bowl and add the avocado and mango. Drizzle the vinaigrette over the salad and top with the slices of smoked chicken. Serve immediately.

Serves 4; 3 portions fruit, 2 portions vegetables

Smoky Joes

1. Pierce the stalk end of the aubergines with a fork. Place on a grill rack and grill for 30 minutes, turning several times, until the skin is blackened and charred all over. Cool slightly, then peel off the skin. Chop the aubergine flesh and set aside.

2. Heat 1 tablespoon of the oil in a frying pan, add the courgette sticks and fry for 5 minutes until tender. Lift out of the pan with a slotted spoon.

3. Heat the remaining oil in the pan, add the onion and garlic, and fry for 5 minutes until softened. Add the aubergine and heat through.

4. Warm the tortillas according to pack directions.

5. Drain the red kidney beans and add to the aubergine mixture with the chilli sauce and chopped coriander. Heat through and season with salt and pepper to taste.

6. Spoon the shredded lettuce, grated cheese, aubergine mixture and courgette sticks on to the tortillas. Roll up and serve, garnished with lime wedges and coriander sprigs.

Serves 2; 7 portions vegetables

2 small aubergines, about 500 g (1 lb) in total
2 tablespoons olive oil
2 small courgettes, about 300 g (10 oz), cut into sticks
1 onion, finely chopped
1 garlic clove, crushed
6 small flour tortillas
210 g (7½ oz) can red kidney beans
1 teaspoon hot chilli sauce, or to taste
3 tablespoons chopped fresh coriander
1 Little Gem lettuce, shredded
1 tablespoon grated mild Cheddar cheese
salt and pepper

To garnish:
lime wedges, coriander sprigs

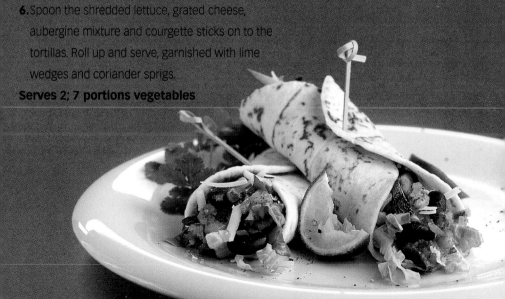

Tomato and vegetable pasta sauce

2 teaspoons olive oil
1 small onion, finely chopped
1 small garlic clove, crushed
100 g (3½ oz) carrot, diced
250 g (8 oz) mixed prepared
  vegetables, such as red pepper,
  courgette, green beans, celery,
  mushrooms, butternut squash,
  diced
200 g (7 oz) can peeled plum
  tomatoes
large pinch of dried marjoram or
  oregano
175 g (6 oz) pasta shapes, such
  as shells or twists
salt and pepper
grated Cheddar cheese,
  to serve

1. Heat the oil in a pan, add the onion and fry for 4–5 minutes, stirring occasionally, until lightly browned. Add the garlic and vegetables and fry for 2 minutes. Stir in the tomatoes and dried herbs with a spoon. Simmer uncovered for 5 minutes, stirring occasionally.

2. Meanwhile, add the pasta to a pan of boiling water and cook for 8–10 minutes until al dente – tender but firm to the bite.

3. Purée the tomato mixture in a blender or processor until smooth, then return to the pan. Reheat if necessary and season to taste.

4. Drain the pasta, rinse with boiling water and drain again. Add to the sauce, toss well, then spoon into serving bowls. Sprinkle each portion with a little grated cheese.

Serves 2; 4 portions vegetables

Tip: Flavour the sauce with a few sprigs of fresh herbs from the garden if available – such as basil or marjoram, or a mixture of herbs.

Pumpkin, garlic and peanut butter soup

1. Place the garlic cloves in a small baking tin and toss with 1 tablespoon of the oil. Place in a preheated oven, 180° (350°F), gas mark 5. Cook for 15–20 minutes until softened. Leave to cool. When cool enough to handle, pop the soft flesh out of the skins and reserve.

2. Heat the remaining oil in a large, heavy-based pan, add the onion, celery and leek and cook gently for 8–10 minutes until softened. Add all the remaining ingredients, including the baked garlic cloves, bring to the boil and simmer for 20–30 minutes until the vegetables are soft. Remove the bayleaf and thyme.

3. Purée the soup in a liquidizer, in batches if necessary. Strain through a sieve, return to the pan and bring back to the boil. Serve with a spoonful of soured cream or crème fraîche in each bowl, accompanied by crusty bread.

Serves 4–6; 5 portions vegetables

6–8 garlic cloves, unpeeled
3 tablespoons olive oil
1 large onion, chopped
2 celery sticks, chopped
1 leek, chopped
6 allspice berries, crushed
1 thyme sprig
1 bayleaf
2 tomatoes, skinned and chopped
50 g (2 oz) peanut butter
750 g (1½ lb) peeled pumpkin, cubed
1.5 litres (2½ pints) chicken stock
salt and pepper
200 ml (7 fl oz) soured cream or crème fraîche, to serve

Cashew nut and oriental vegetable stir-fry

2 tablespoons vegetable oil
1 green pepper, deseeded and
 finely sliced
2 red peppers, deseeded and
 finely sliced
1 red onion, finely sliced
2 carrots, peeled and sliced or
 cut into strips
125 g (4 oz) pak choi or green
 cabbage, shredded
175 g (6 oz) beansprouts
2 tablespoons oyster sauce
2 tablespoons hoisin sauce
2–3 tablespoons soy sauce or
 tamari
5 tablespoons water
75 g (3 oz) cashew nuts, toasted
1 tablespoon sesame seeds,
 toasted
handful of coriander leaves
brown rice or noodles,
 to serve

1. Heat the oil in a wok or large frying pan, and when very hot add the green and red peppers, red onion, carrots, pak choi and beansprouts. Stir-fry over a high heat for 3–4 minutes or until piping hot.

2. Mix the oyster, hoisin and soy sauces with the water and add to the pan. Stir-fry the mixture for a further minute.

3. Add the cashew nuts and sesame seeds and toss together. Add the coriander leaves, and serve immediately with brown rice or noodles.

Serves 4–6; 8 portions vegetables

Grilled tropical fruit

1. Cut the mango lengthways, either side of the stone, then cut the flesh from the skin into chunky pieces. Halve the papaya, scoop out the seeds, then peel and cut the flesh into wedges. Cut the skin from the pineapple, then quarter it lengthways and cut out the core. Cut the pineapple flesh into smaller wedges. Peel and quarter the kiwi fruit.

2. Line a grill pan with foil, bringing the foil up over the side of the pan to contain the juices. Arrange the fruit in the pan in a single layer. Brush with the butter and spoon over the ginger syrup.

3. Thinly slice the stem ginger, then cut each slice into thin slivers. Scatter over the fruit and grill for about 5 minutes until the fruit are beginning to colour. Transfer to serving bowls, adding any juices from the pan.

4. Halve the passion fruit, scoop out the pulp and spoon over the warm fruit salad to serve.

Serves 4; 7 portions fruit

1 large mango
1 papaya
1 small pineapple
2 kiwi fruit
25 g (1 oz) unsalted butter, melted
1 piece preserved stem ginger, plus 2 tablespoons syrup from the jar
2 passion fruit

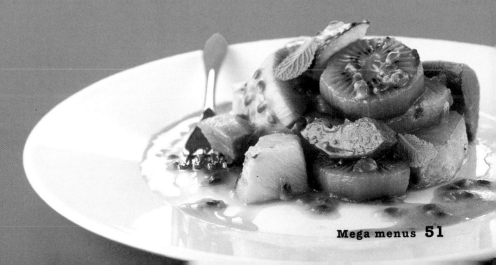

Super smoothies

These tasty treats provide an easy way to bump up your portions. For recipes including ice, make sure you use a blender that is suitable for crushing ice.

Banana smoothie with tofu

300 g (10 oz) tofu
2 bananas
1 litre (1¾ pints) white grape or apple juice
2 teaspoons linseeds

1. Roughly chop the tofu and banana and put them into a food processor or blender with half of the fruit juice. Blend until smooth. Roughly grind the linseeds in a coffee grinder, or use a pestle and mortar, then add to the smoothie with the remaining fruit juice and blend until smooth. Serve immediately.

Serves 4; 3 portions fruit

Peach, pear and raspberry smoothie

1 ripe peach
1 ripe dessert pear
125 g (4 oz) raspberries
200 ml (7 fl oz) peach juice
250 ml (8 fl oz) crushed ice
pear slices, to decorate (optional)

1. Roughly chop the peach and pear and put into a food processor or blender. Add the remaining ingredients and blend until smooth. Serve decorated with a pear slice, if you like.

Serves 2–3; 3 portions fruit

Fruity beauty

half an avocado
1 frozen banana
1 cup strawberries, hulled
splash of soya milk
pinch of cardamom

1.Roughly chop the avocado and banana and put into a food processor or blender. Add the remaining ingredients and blend until smooth and creamy. Serve immediately.

Serves 1; 3 portions fruit

Berry nice

2 bananas
1 cup raspberries
1 cup blueberries
1 small glass cranberry juice

1.Roughly chop the bananas and put into a food processor or blender. Add the berries and pour in the cranberry juice. Blend until smooth and creamy. For a thicker, creamier drink you can also add 2 tablespoons of natural yogurt.

Serves 1; 5 portions fruit

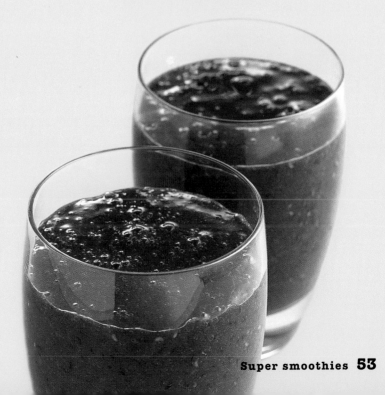

Papaya, melon and strawberry smoothie

1 papaya, peeled, deseeded
  and quartered
250 g (8 oz) honeydew melon,
  roughly chopped
6 large strawberries, hulled
150 ml (5 fl oz) coconut milk
sugar, to taste
crushed ice, to serve

1. Place the papaya and melon in a food processor or blender and process until smooth. Add the strawberries, blend, and then add the coconut milk. Add sugar according to taste, and serve in glasses over crushed ice.

Serves 3; 3 portions fruit

Mango magic

half a mango
1 slice watermelon
1 cup blueberries or blackberries
1 cup frozen orange juice

1. Roughly chop the mango and watermelon and put into a blender or food processor with the the blueberries and frozen orange juice. Blend until smooth and creamy.

Serves 1; 4 portions fruit

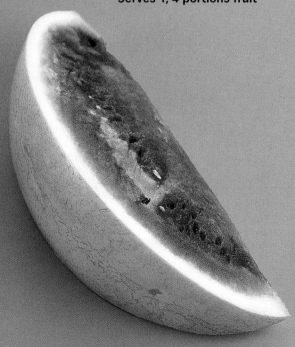

Eat 5 for kids

Eating fruit and vegetables is important at any age in our lives, but for children it's vital. In the short term, it provides the essential nutrients they need for strong, healthy growth. Between 1–6 months and 1–6 years of age, a child's weight should quadruple, and once a child reaches adolescence the changes puberty brings means their nutrient needs reach adulthood before they do. But fruit and vegetables are also important for long-term health; and **the earlier you start eating a healthy diet the greater your foundation for a long life and a healthy old age**.

The problem, however, is that kids and vegetables don't always mix. Whether it's a 2-year-old who has decided that broccoli is evil or a teenager who jumps from one fast-food fix to the next, it can be hard to get children to eat fruit and vegetables. Hard doesn't mean impossible, though. Increasingly, experts are looking into why kids don't eat fruit and vegetables and coming up with new ways to make the whole process easier.

Over the next 6 pages, there is plenty of advice on how to persuade your child – whatever age – that Eating 5 is not only good for them but can also be fun.

Babies

Young babies get all the nutrition they need from milk, so the Eat 5 programme is not relevant for them. When you wean them on to solids, however, you need to focus on small portions of nutritious foods (including some fruit and vegetables) but not aim to force-feed endless portions.

Just one word of advice: researchers believe that some food allergies occur when a child is exposed to certain foods too early. They recommend that citrus fruit, berries and tomatoes should not be given to a baby until it is over 1 year old. Also foods with tough skins, like grapes, or that are very chewy, like carrots, need to be mashed or chopped for the under-3s to minimize the risk of choking.

Toddlers

When it comes to fruit and vegetables and toddlers, there are 2 main problems. The first is that, like the rest of their bodies, toddlers' stomachs are extremely small. This means that while toddlers are still recommended to eat 5 portions of fruit and vegetables a day the amounts in each portion are much less than needed by adults. As a simple rule, be guided by the quantity the child can hold in one hand and aim to serve that amount as a portion – and as the hand grows, so should the portion. Many people don't understand this and serve much larger portions that children can't eat. This can lead to 1 of 2 things: a negative reaction in the child to the sight of a pile of fruit or vegetables, meaning they won't eat them; or kids who clean their plate when they don't need to, and suffer the consequences. Obesity in children under 4 is now at record levels – in the UK alone, a third of children under 4 are overweight and 1 in 10 is obese. Knowing the correct size of fruit and vegetable portions to help your child eat correctly is vital to get them to benefit from Eating 5.

You also need to note that, while adults are advised to focus more of their portions on vegetables than fruit, for children it's the other way round, as they need the natural sugars and increased calories per portion that fruit provides over vegetables. Ideally they should eat 3 portions of fruit and 2 of vegetables and you should spread the portions over 5–7 small meals and snacks a day.

The second problem with produce and pre-schoolers is that toddlers may have teeth but that doesn't mean they can chew everything adults can. A lot of foods are still too tough for them to deal with comfortably – a raw carrot, if it's not cut into a small enough portion, can be a mammoth task. Mashing foods can help here – as can making sure things are served in bite-sized pieces. Toddlers also have a low attention span when it comes to food – there are too many other things to discover.

You must choose those foods carefully, though. The biggest problem for parents of toddlers is that their children often don't like many fruit and vegetables. Sometimes this is just a case of the 'terrible 2s', but often there's a scientific explanation. **Toddlers have more tastebuds than adults, not just on their tongue but also in the lining of their cheeks and the roof of their mouth, meaning that younger children taste fruit and vegetables very differently from the rest of us.** Dark green leafy and cruciferous vegetables taste bitter, and citrus fruit and tart berries like cranberries taste sharp and sour. Trying to force-feed a child particular fruit or vegetables if they don't like them can therefore be a very unrewarding experience for both parties. If a child dislikes a fruit or vegetable, don't force them to eat it – it can set up a negative cycle for all fruit and vegetables. Instead, focus on sweeter, creamier fruit and vegetables like bananas, avocados, pumpkin, sweet potatoes, carrots, strawberries, sweetcorn and peas. When you do cook the more bitter varieties for your child, serve them with a little dairy produce – spinach mixed with a little ricotta cheese, for example – as this will soften the taste on the tongue.

School children

When children start school, the barriers they put up tend to be more psychological – and the techniques you need to employ to help your child fit to the Eat 5 plan need to be similarly mental.

To start with, *fruit and vegetables need to be made fun.* Studies by food educators Food Groupie have shown that children who understand what fruit and vegetables are, where they come from and what they do for you are more likely to eat fruit and vegetables than those who are just told they have to have them. Having children involved in cooking, preparing and growing of fruit and vegetables (even something as simple as a tomato plant) helps here; or, if it's a feasible alternative, take them to farms or pick-your-own orchards so they become involved in the process.

You're also up against a lot of peer pressure with this age of child; they want to fit in with what the other kids are eating (or think they should be). Keeping foods interesting will help here. For smaller children, this can be as simple as cutting fruit and vegetables into shapes with cookie-cutters, or using vegetables to make pictures or shapes on the plate. With older children, it can mean choosing 'sophisticated' foods like wraps or smoothies (see pages 45 and 52–54), which they find interesting and cool. As a general rule, look at the adverts on television that are selling 'fast' or less nutritious foods to your child and ask how you can incorporate those serving techniques into your cooking.

Of course none of this will work if, again, you are trying to get kids to eat more food than they can comfortably handle. Studies from the Children's Hospital in

Portions for school children

For children aged 5–11, a portion of fruit or vegetables is the equivalent amount that would fill half a cup, with 3 of the recommended 5 portions coming from fruit.

The rainbow rules

Making the eating of fruit and vegetables into a game can be effective. An easy way to do this is to integrate the rainbow rules. The idea is that every day the child has to try to eat 5 different colours of fruit and vegetables. To make this more fun, encourage them to cut pictures of fruit and vegetables from magazines (or draw them). Now make a chart of all the different colours of vegetables there are (red, yellow, green, purple, white and orange), and every time they eat a vegetable of a colour they should stick a picture on the chart. The idea is to stick as many pictures on the chart each week as possible. Similar games, like picking 2 of each colour in the supermarket, also helps to get children involved.

Columbus, Ohio, showed that children of this age generally eat 67 per cent of any meal – and fruit and vegetables tend to be left behind. Making main dishes like meat or pizza smaller will tip the balance so more fruit and vegetables will be consumed.

What about making them eat foods they don't like? Here parents need to make a decision. Is it a true dislike, or caused because their newest school friend doesn't like carrots? If it's a true dislike, it may be better to avoid that food and focus on nutrients elsewhere. If it's a passing fad, or if a child suddenly decides they hate all fruit and vegetables, it's OK to use subterfuge – grate foods into soups and stews, mash hated foods into potatoes, supply dips with fresh vegetables or fruit, use dairy products to disguise more bitter tastes, and use jelly to cover a variety of fresh fruit. Also remember that children learn by example – if you're eating only French fries with your steak, why should they eat a portion of green beans too?

Teenagers

The last stage of childhood development can often be the most frustrating to parents. At an age when children can truly understand the benefits of good nutrition on their health, they have a tendency to enter a world of fast-food fixes and faddy diets which bear no relation to what's good for them.

The problem is that *85 per cent of teenagers don't reach anywhere near the recommended intake of fruit and vegetables.* They like to snack, but snack heavy meal patterns may make it harder for them to get fruit and vegetables unless they are persuaded to think of them as foods they can grab on the go. Worries about losing weight make skipping meals common for girls, and worries about gaining weight may mean boys skip fruit and vegetables in favour of portions of protein they feel will help boost their bulk. The fact that fruit and vegetables aren't marketed in the way fast food is means that they just aren't programmed to think of fresh foods first.

The vegetarian teenager

Parents who may think they don't need to worry are those whose children decide in their teens to go vegetarian. Don't be so sure, because many vegetarian teens eat nutritionally poorly, swapping meat for high-fat dairy products and foregoing vegetables completely. If your child is vegetarian, generally they should base their daily diet around 8–10 portions of carbohydrates like rice, pasta, potatoes or bread. They should remember to include 2–3 servings of a variety of protein-rich foods every day, such as nuts, beans and legumes, cheese, eggs and products such as tofu or tvp (textured vegetable protein). Then they should aim for 3 portions of dairy and at least 5 fruits and vegetables a day. Use the tips given here to try to ensure this happens, and remember that if it's eaten well, a vegetarian diet can rival that of a meat-eater in terms of all nutrients.

How do you overcome these problems? You need to help kids live their own lives – but make the right choices. The first step is to give teens the nutritional information they need. Explaining to a teenage girl accurately why skipping meals slows the metabolism, preventing weight loss, and the difference in calories between an apple and a chocolate bar may encourage healthy choices. With boys, explaining how different vitamins and minerals work in terms of growth can help. For both sexes, talking through how fruit and vegetables help hair and skin can help to focus the mind. Just make sure that the information you give *is* accurate (use the internet or buy some good nutrition books); there's nothing worse than telling them, for example, that sugar causes spots (it doesn't) and then having them find out it's not true.

Adapt your shopping and meal habits to fit in with your teens. **The average teenager eats 7 snacks in the day and 3 in the evening.** The traditional 3 sit-down meals just doesn't apply to them. If your fridge is stocked with grabbable snacks – again, those with a cool image like smoothies or exotic fruit like mangos – your children are as likely to choose those as any other snack. When teens do eat with the family, give them a choice of 2 or 3 vegetables to eat – when schools in Ohio did this, fruit and vegetable consumption went up by 17 per cent. Even ask them what fruit and vegetables they'd *like* to eat, and buy these. Teens tend to reject all they associate with their parents – by giving them produce that's just for them you tap into that desire for non-conformity. Ignore them wanting to eat bizarre foods at odd times – if they want cold vegetarian pizza for breakfast and fruit salad for dinner, let it happen. What matters is that they eat the nutrients, not *when* they eat them. If all else fails, remember you probably went through exactly the same thing.

Eat 5 for pregnant women

What you eat when you're expecting is one of the most important nutrition decisions you need to make in life. The nutrients you take in are what feed your baby. The more you give them the happier and healthier you both will be, and not just while you are pregnant, either. Research now seems to point to the idea that what their mother ate while pregnant determines a person's health throughout their lives, with babies born to mothers with low levels of nutrients in their diets having the highest risk of heart disease, finding learning most difficult and even being less likely to marry in later life.

The good news is that good pregnancy nutrition does not have to be hard. When you're pregnant, your body absorbs a higher proportion of nutrients from food, so that everything you eat works harder. However, even with this internal boost, the increased need for most nutrients that you have in pregnancy means many doctors recommend that eating 5 each day is especially important. The reason is that fruit and vegetables help you get high doses of the following, as well as providing fibre, which can help beat problems such as constipation.

Folic acid

This is the most important thing you as a mother-to-be can take in, as it's been shown to reduce the risk of birth defects like spina bifida. Pregnant women – and those trying to conceive – are recommended to get around 600 mcg of folic acid daily. Aim for at least 2 portions of folate-rich foods (dark green leafy vegetables, beans and chickpeas, asparagus) daily and supplement these further with a 400 mcg folic acid supplement.

Vitamin C

A low vitamin C intake during pregnancy has been linked to a higher incidence of premature birth. If you add to this the fact that vitamin C is used by our bodies to help in the formation of new tissues, and that it helps boost the absorption of iron (another vital natal nutrient), you can see why the average woman needs 25 per cent more vitamin C when she's pregnant than normal. You'll get this by using at least 1 of your fruit and vegetable portions on high vitamin C foods like half a guava, 2 tablespoons of red peppers or 2 kiwi fruit.

Beta-carotene

Vitamin A is needed to help the baby develop the respiratory, gastrointestinal and urinary systems, but taken 'neat' it can actually cause birth defects. This is where fruit and vegetables come in. As explained before, fruit and vegetables contain beta-carotene which your body converts into vitamin A, and this form is not related to birth defects. Aim for at least 2 portions of green, yellow or orange fruit or vegetables daily.

Calcium

Growing a healthy bone structure is such an important part of your child's development that if you're not getting enough calcium in your diet the baby will actually start to draw calcium from your bones, softening them. While the majority of your calcium should be provided by the recommended 4 portions of dairy products a day, you can also boost levels with calcium-rich vegetables like broccoli and kale.

When sickness strikes

Some women find green vegetables trigger sickness in the first trimester. One reason for this is thought to be a higher sensitivity to bitter tastes in the leaves. If you do experience this, skip the vegetables that are causing your nausea and focus on other types, and fruit. Your doctor may also prescribe a multi-vitamin supplement, so seek advice.

Eat 5 for the elderly

Our needs for fruit and vegetables also alter as we get older and we need to eat a diet more dense in nutrients than when we were younger. As we age so do the body's processes, and the efficiency with which digestive enzymes and processes work may begin to decline. Obviously, the higher in nutrients your diet is in the first place the less chance there is of this happening – plus, by focusing on fruit and vegetables that actually promote a healthy digestive system (papaya and pineapple, for example, both contain enzymes vital for the digestion process) you can help boost your intake.

There's also the fact that a slowing metabolism means the average 70-year-old requires 10 per cent fewer calories than someone 40 years younger to maintain their weight. Because this means you can eat less food without suffering the consequences of weight gain, it's important to choose foods that are high in nutrients and low in calories – like fruit and vegetables.

Fruit and vegetables also provide high levels of water. Even as young as 40, our ability to determine when we are thirsty diminishes. This is not good as 70 per cent of our bodies is water and we need it to function correctly. By providing water, fruit and vegetables can help slow the mental and physical slowdown that can be attributed to dehydration – and stave off more serious problems. According to US health insurer Medicare, dehydration is among the most common reasons why elderly patients are admitted to hospital – and half those of those over 65 admitted to hospital with diseases accompanied by dehydration die within a year.

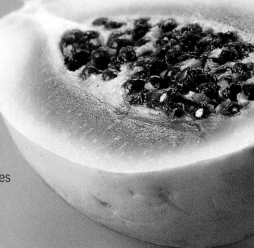

As well as aiding your general health, fruit and vegetables may help slow down some of the main processes of ageing. They can't work miracles –

although they have been demonstrated to have major effects in the prevention of age-related problems such as cancer and heart disease, doctors generally say that they need to be introduced into the diet before you hit 40 to make a real difference. But some things can be helped, as described below.

Eyesight

Research by one ophthalmologist in Chicago found that eating a 150 g (5 oz) portion of spinach every day actually improved the vision of his macular-degeneration patients in just 3 months.

Cholesterol

It's one of the major risk factors for heart disease, yet studies have shown that many foods can help reduce its presence in the blood in a matter of weeks. For example, French researchers who asked 30 middle-aged adults to consume 2–3 apples a day for a month found half had their cholesterol levels decrease by as much as 29 per cent. Other good cholesterol lowerers are carrots, avocados and beans.

Memory loss

Animal studies have shown that supplementing the diet for 8 weeks with blueberry extract improved loss of memory and loss of balance that affect the elderly. Aim for at least 1 cup of fresh fruit a day.

So what does this mean to you? While 5 should be the minimum number of fruit and vegetable portions you get in a day, to live life to the maximum in your golden years you should try to improve on this. Remember, frozen and canned vegetables do count, so you don't need to be concerned about fresh foods going off. Also, the heat processing of these foods often makes them softer to eat – one of the main concerns for those whose teeth just aren't quite as good (or as natural) as they once were. Finally, take time to experiment. Our sense of taste changes as we age, and so fruit and vegetables that were too sharp or too bitter for you when you were young may now taste just right – make this the time to find out.

Questions and answers

Now you should know just about everything about the whys and wherefores of eating 5. Just in case anything has been overlooked, however, here are the answers to some common questions.

Q: **Are organic vegetables more nutritious than non-organic?**
A: According to research by British organic group The Soil Association, organic vegetables do contain slightly higher levels of minerals like calcium, potassium, iron and zinc. A small study published in the journal *Nature* in 2001 found that in blind taste tests organic vegetables did have more intense tastes than non-organically farmed produce, which may also make you more likely to eat them.

Q: **I'm scared about the effects of pesticides on my body but can't afford to go organic. Which produce is most likely to be affected by pesticides?**
A: According to the British Soil Association, at the highest risk of contamination are squashy fruit like strawberries or blackberries, which absorb pesticides more readily than harder fruit. Salad crops can also be a problem, as they are heavily treated – some lettuce crops are sprayed 15 times while they grow. In the USA, the Food and Drug Administration also ranked bell peppers, spinach, cherries, apples and peaches as potentially high-risk foods. Switching to organic versions of these could therefore allay your fears. For other fruit and vegetables, cleaning may help.

Q: **Do I need to scrub fruit and vegetables before I eat them?**
A: It's best to. As well as the pesticide issue, dirt on fruit and vegetables can contain bacteria like salmonella or E.coli, which could cause food poisoning. The best way to debug (and reduce pesticide count) on fresh foods is to wash them under running water and use a small vegetable (or nail) brush to scrub the skins. You should even do this before cutting fruit where you don't eat the peel (like pineapple or melon), or you may

transfer pesticides or bacteria into the fruit on the blade of the knife. Mould also carries bacteria, so throw away any mouldy fruit or vegetables.

Q: I don't really like the taste of most fruit and vegetables. What should I do?

A: According to the Taste Laboratory at Yale University in the USA, the reason some people don't like fruit and vegetables is that they are so-called supertasters who have more than the average number of tastebuds on their tongue. This causes you to pick on bitter tastes in many fruit and vegetables (particularly cruciferous vegetables like cabbage) that other people can't taste. This doesn't mean, however, that all fruit and vegetables will taste bad to you – sweet or creamy-tasting produce like carrots, melons, avocados, strawberries, tomatoes, coconuts and bell peppers should all still taste good. You can also drop bitter vegetables like brussels sprouts and cabbage into boiling salted water for 1 minute before serving which cuts the bitter taste, or add a dash or lemon which counteracts the bitter taste without adding salt.

Q: Is it better to eat fruit and vegetables in season?

A: Yes. Vegetables sold in season are more likely to have been grown locally, so will potentially have spent less time in transit than winter strawberries flown in from the other side of the world. This means they could contain higher levels of nutrients. If you want to eat out-of-season vegetables, always choose the ripest looking – or choose frozen or canned varieties which may have lost fewer nutrients than fresh.

Q: I live alone and fresh fruit and vegetables go off quickly. Can I do anything to make them last longer?

A: Choosing ripe, unbruised produce will help extend the life of your food, but basically it all comes down to storage. Keep them in the fridge – ideally at 2°C (36°F). Put them in the salad drawer, as this is the coldest part of the fridge. Don't put them near the door, as this actually warms up a little every time the door is opened, and changes in temperature increase vitamin loss. Chop fruit and vegetables just before you use them, and keep any cut produce in airtight containers or ideally in sealed, vacuum-packed bags – oxygen destroys the nutrients and makes foods go off quicker.

Q: Someone said drinking tea with meals cancels out nutrients in fruit and vegetables. Is this true?

A: Partly. The nutrient in question is iron, which is found in dark green leafy vegetables. According to information in the *Journal of the Vegetarian Resource Group*, tannins in tea and caffeine in coffee actually reduce the amount of iron you absorb from foods by up to 65 per cent. In fact, coffee has even been shown to do this if you drink it up to an hour after eating. Skip both when eating iron-rich foods, and switch to orange juice (or any other food or drink high in vitamin C) as this increases the amount of iron you absorb.

Q: Why does juice only count once a day?

A: Because, while it contains vitamins and minerals, juice doesn't contain the fibre we also need for health. Smoothies are slightly different, as the whole fruit tends to be used, so fibre is present.

Q: Does it matter if I eat the same 5 fruit and vegetables every day?

A: It's better than not eating any – and, so long as you are mixing and matching your colours, you're probably not going to do much harm. However, according to Dr Adam Drewnowski at the University of Washington, for optimum health you should eat 16 different foodstuffs (including meat, fish and starchy foods) every 3 days, so try for as varied a diet as possible.

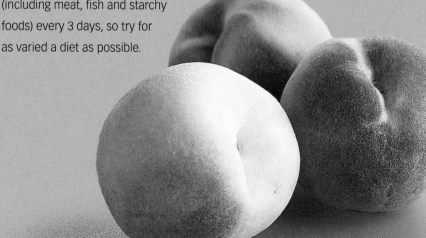

Q: Beans and cruciferous vegetables upset my stomach. How can I build them into a healthy diet without feeling uncomfortable?

A: The gas that some people experience when they eat these vegetables occurs because the body finds it hard to break down sugar within them. It doesn't mean they need be taken off the menu, though. In India, it's been found that adding garlic or ginger to the cooking water helps break down the sugars naturally and therefore prevent problems. In the case of beans, the US Department of Agriculture recommends rinsing beans 3 or 4 times in fresh water before you start cooking them. This also seems to break down some of the sugars. If you still get gas attacks, peppermint tea will help to naturally deflate your system.

Q: How can I tell if a prepared food counts as a portion?

A: The ingredient list is the big giveaway. Ingredients in a food have to be listed in order of the amount used in the food. If a single fruit or vegetable (like the strawberry in a strawberry yogurt) isn't first on the list, or if more than 3 vegetables or fruit don't appear in the top 5 or 6 ingredients in a combination dish (like a curry or lasagne), then it probably doesn't count. Also, look at how much of the food you eat – while tomatoes may be the top ingredient in ketchup, the fact that you only eat a teaspoon means it doesn't count.

Q: I've heard that high doses of vitamin C are bad for you. Does this mean that if I eat more than 5 portions I put my health at risk?

A: No. The amounts in studies that show negative effects of the nutrients in fruit and vegetables were much higher than can be delivered by the daily diet – even if you eat 10 or 15 portions of fruit and vegetables. The only thing that will happen by eating more fruit and vegetables is that you get more health benefits.

Q: I have a really busy job and some days it's impossible for me to reach my 5 portions – if I only manage 2 one day, can I eat 7 the next?

A: Yes. Researchers who compile the food pyramids that show healthy-eating guidelines say that the amounts are cumulative. However, it is best to try to keep your levels constant, as the body can only store certain levels of many nutrients (including the B vitamins and vitamin C) in one go, so flooding your body one day and depriving it the next may not provide you with optimum nutrient levels. If you are busy, planning ahead can really help – refer to the snacks section (see page 44).

Q: Can fatty fruit like avocados, coconuts and olives really be good for me?

A: Strange, but true. Because avocados and olives actually contain high levels of healthy mono-unsaturated fats, they benefit your heart rather than harm it. In fact, studies from Australia have shown that women who ate avocados daily for 3 weeks actually lowered cholesterol better than those sticking to a low-fat diet. Both avocados and olives also contain anti-oxidants and other cancer-fighting phytonutrients. Coconuts are a slightly different matter. They contain the saturated fat that is linked to heart disease, but research is showing they do have other health-promoting properties, including immune-boosting properties and the ability to help stop alcohol damaging the liver. So, while they shouldn't be a daily diet staple, for a tasty treat they are fine.

Q: Do vegetable sauces, salsas or dips count?

A: Yes. With fresh tomato- or vegetable-based pasta sauces, salsas or vegetable-based dips, half a cupful counts as 1 portion.

Q: Do ready-made vegetarian meals count?

A: Vegetarian meals – vegetable-heavy meals like vegetarian curries, soups or lasagne – count as 1 portion, so long as at least 2 tablespoons of vegetables have been used in the preparation.

Q: Can't I get all this from a pill?

A: The simple answer is yes, but in fact it's not really simple. Over the last few years, supplement companies have been bringing out tablets containing the vital health-boosting ingredients, such as anti-oxidants, phytoestrogens and bioflavonoids, that are contained in fruit and vegetables. However, although researchers *think* it's the specific phytonutrients like the flavonoids or beta-carotene that are acting positively on our bodies, they don't know for sure – nor do they know if other ingredients in fruit and vegetables work with the flavonoids or the anti-oxidants to enable them to function. This was shown recently by the results of a trial by the American Institute for Cancer Research who looked at 22,000 male doctors and found those taking beta-carotene supplements had no decreased incidence of cancer at all. This is a very different picture from that of people eating foods high in beta-carotene who have considerably lower risk of a whole of host of cancers.

In fact, supplementing with individual phytonutrients may even cause you harm. Studies in 1994 and 1996 found smokers who took high-dose supplements of beta-carotene (in a study supposed to show how the nutrient protected them) actually had a higher risk of lung cancer than those not popping the pills. Nowadays, researchers think they know why – it seems that, while the low doses of beta-carotene we get from our diet protect the lungs, high doses attack protective chemicals in the body and switch on proteins that cause cells to divide – making cell mutations that lead to cancers more likely. The truth is that most of the studies showing protective benefits for phytonutrients demonstrate that they have occurred when the nutrients have been delivered in their natural form. This leads researchers to believe either that all the nutrients work together to provide this protective package, so won't work alone in supplement form, or that the protection is being carried out in the 3,800 phytonutrients that nobody has really investigated yet. Whatever the reason, however, one thing is clear. Supplements are not a substitute for 5 portions of fruit and vegetables a day. If you want to take them, do; but stick to a good 'one a day' type of multi-vitamin and mineral supplement (rather than aiming for individual vitamins or nutrients), and use them just as the name suggests, as a supplement to your healthy-eating plan, and all will be well.

Q: **Do I need more nutrients?**

A: You don't have to be pregnant or old to need different levels of certain nutrients, anything from your weekend activities to your eye colour can determine which nutrients you really need.

If you have blue or green eyes: Make at least 1 of your 5 daily portions a lutein-containing food like spinach, kale or broccoli. Studies at Johns Hopkins University School of Medicine in Baltimore found that people with blue or green eyes actually find it harder to absorb lutein than those with brown eyes, and may therefore be at higher risk of age-related macular degeneration.

If you're starting an exercise programme: When we exercise, the body produces free radicals. These harmful substances, thought to increase heart disease, actually go up when you work out. While studies show that the fitter you get the better your body copes with them, when you start an exercise programme (or even if you're a weekend exerciser who does nothing all week) this system doesn't react as well – meaning you could be more prone to injury and aches (which are often caused by free radicals attacking muscles). Therefore, help your body by increasing your intake of vitamin C and beta-carotene based vegetables. At present, there's no recommended level for this, but adding 2 portions a day to your Eat 5 programme is probably a safe bet.

If you're a smoker: Smoking 20 cigarettes a day depletes the amount of vitamin C in your body by 40 per cent. Therefore, if you really must smoke, you need to boost your intake of vitamin C foods. Aim for at least 3 portions of high vitamin C foods a day (on top of your 5) – and make sure 1 of those comes from orange or another citrus juice. Research by the US Horticultural Research Laboratory in Fort Pierce, Florida, has shown that citrus fruit juice has the ability to switch off the enzyme in the body that causes some ingredients in cigarette smoke to turn cancerous.

If you're quitting smoking: Focusing your diet on fruit and vegetables could help you beat the cravings. According to UK support group QUIT, the presence of alkaline foods (like fruit and vegetables) in your system slows the rate at which nicotine leaves the system. This means you get fewer withdrawal symptoms, making it easier to beat the habit. When you're quitting, include at least 1 portion of fruit or vegetables at every meal, and keep fruit or vegetable snacks to hand.

If you're going through the menopause: Increasing your intake of phytoestrogen-containing vegetables (like alfalfa sprouts and endame) can help reduce menopause symptoms. In a study at Bowman Gray University in North Carolina, women eating 20 g (1 oz) of soya protein a day had lower incidence of hot flushes. Also, the cholesterol levels in their blood decreased. Aim for 1 portion of a phytoestrogen-rich food a day as part of your Eat 5 regime.

If you have diabetes: Choosing fruit and vegetables with a particularly high fibre content is important. Fibre has the ability to help regulate sugar levels in the blood. In studies published in the *New England Journal of Medicine*, people with type 2 diabetes who increased their fibre intake to 50 g (2 oz) a day (using 7–8 portions of fruit and vegetables a day, and focused on high-fibre choices like papaya, courgettes and oranges) developed more stable glucose levels. Ask your doctor for advice on whether this could be a good approach for you.

At a glance

This quick guide will show you, at a glance, which beneficial nutrients your favourite fruit and vegetables contain. It also gives a brief outline of the health benefits associated with each of them.

Alfalfa
High in: vitamin C, folate, beta-carotene, vitamin B5, phytoestrogens
Good for: reducing menopausal symptoms, bone health, shown to fight leukaemia cells

Apples
High in: fibre, vitamin C, folic acid, iron, the flavonoid quercetin
Good for: cholesterol fighting, lung strengthening, anti-carcinogenic

Apricots
High in: fibre, vitamin C, beta-carotene, calcium, phosphorus, iron, the carotenoid lycopene

Good for: constipation, bone health, anaemia, immunity

Asparagus
High in: fibre, B vitamins (including folic acid), vitamin C, magnesium, copper, potassium, detoxifying glucosinolates
Good for: strengthening veins and capillaries, positive liver function, said to be anti-cancer, controls blood pressure

Avocados
High in: B vitamins, vitamin E, folic acid, the carotenoid lutein, the detoxifier glutathione
Good for: cholesterol lowering, heart health, eyesight, skin. Seem to have a preventive effect on prostate cancer

Bananas
High in: fibre, vitamin C, B vitamins (particularly B6), potassium, magnesium
Good for: stress relief, energy boosting, blood pressure control, improving mood

Beans
High in: fibre, B vitamins, calcium, iron, potassium, phosphorus, zinc, plant sterols
Good for: energy provision, diabetes, fighting cholesterol, controlling blood pressure

Beetroot
High in: vitamin C, beta-carotene, folic acid, iron, phosphorus, sodium, magnesium, the anti-oxidant beta-cyanin
Good for: energy, anaemia, said to have anti-cancer effects, strengthening the liver

Blueberries, bilberries and blackberries
High in: fibre, vitamin C, anti-oxidants known as anthocyanins
Good for: memory loss and anti-ageing, cancer fighting, immunity boosters, fighting urinary tract infections

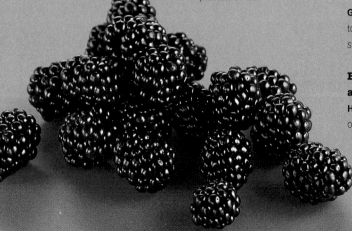

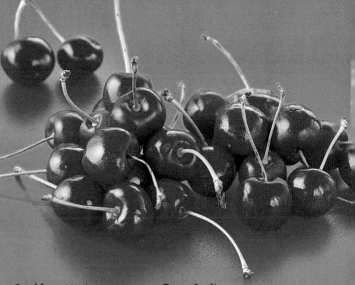

Broccoli
High in: calcium, folate, vitamin C, selenium, the glucosilinate sulforaphane
Good for: bone health, anti-cancer – seems to have particularly strong preventive action for colon and rectal cancers

Brussels sprouts
High in: fibre, vitamin C, beta-carotene, folic acid, the glucosilinate sulforaphane
Good for: stroke prevention, anti-cancer effects particularly digestive and colorectal cancers. May also regulate oestrogen levels thereby lowering breast cancer risk

Cabbages
High in: fibre, vitamin C, beta-carotene, glucosilinates including sulforaphane
Good for: general detoxification and liver function, anti-cancer effects – like many other cruciferous vegetables cabbages act particularly on the stomach

Carrots
High in: fibre, vitamin C, beta-carotene
Good for: fighting blindness, seem to lower lung cancer risk, reducing cholesterol

Cherries
High in: vitamin C, fibre, anti-oxidants known as anthocyanins, various flavonoids

Good for: said to be cancer fighting, insomnia as they promote sleep hormones, contain painkilling properties

Cranberries
High in: vitamin C, folic acid, anti-oxidants known as anthocyanins
Good for: prevention of urinary tract infections, preventing tooth decay, anti-ageing effects

Garlic
High in: the anti-oxidants quercitin and allicin
Good for: strengthening lungs, preventing arterial hardening, anti-bacterial effects, may fight stomach cancer

Globe artichokes
High in: fibre, vitamin C, folate, potassium, magnesium, glucosinolates
Good for: digestion, detoxification, fighting cholesterol

Grapefruit
High in: fibre, beta-carotene, vitamin C, flavonoids including terpene and d-limonene
Good for: general health and immunity

Grapes
High in: fibre, vitamin C, anti-oxidants – particularly revestrol
Good for: thinning the blood and reducing risk of clotting, lowering cholesterol, said to be cancer fighting

Guavas
High in: fibre, vitamin C, beta-carotene, lycopene
Good for: lowering cholesterol, soothing the digestive system

Kiwi fruits
High in: vitamin C, lutein, fibre, copper, potassium and magnesium

Good for: immune boosting, cholesterol lowering, said to be cancer fighting, heart health, eyesight

Lemons
High in: vitamin C, beta-carotene, flavonoids including terpenes and d-limonene
Good for: preventing kidney stones, stimulation of the immune system, energy boosting

Lettuce (dark green or red varieties)
High in: beta-carotene, the carotenoid lutein, folic acid
Good for: general health and nutrient provision, eyesight, insomnia (also contains sleep-inducing ingredients)

Mangoes
High in: fibre, vitamin C, beta-carotene, potassium
Good for: digestion, immune boosting, control of blood pressure and cholesterol

Melons
High in: vitamin C, carotenoids, fibre, potassium
Good for: lowering blood pressure, general health and immunity

Mushrooms (oriental varieties)
High in: B vitamins, vitamin D, essential fatty acids, phytoestrogens

Good for: immunity, bone health, lowering cholesterol, may act against breast cancer

Onions
High in: the flavonoid quercetin
Good for: strengthening the lungs, bone building, heart health, immune boosting

Oranges
High in: B vitamins, vitamin C, flavonoids, specialist anti-oxidants
Good for: immunity, cholesterol lowering and general heart health, said to be anti-cancer

Papayas
High in: fibre, vitamin C, beta-carotene
Good for: digestive system, anti-inflammatory, immune system

Passion fruit
High in: B vitamins, vitamin C, various carotenoids
Good for: general health and immunity, the juice is also slightly sedative helping stress and sleep patterns. May help prevent some gastric cancers

Peas
High in: fibre, vitamin C, beta-carotene, folic acid, zinc, the carotenoids lutein and zeaxanthin
Good for: eyesight, cholesterol, diabetes control

Peppers
High in: vitamin C, beta-carotene, the carotenoid lycopene
Good for: said to be anti-cancer – particularly lung or prostate cancers, heart disease, immunity boosting

Pineapples
High in: fibre, vitamin C, beta-carotene, the flavonoid quercetin
Good for: general all round health and nutrient provision. Also contains bromelain, which helps heal bruising

Plums
High in: fibre, beta-carotene and other anti-oxidants particularly anthocyanins
Good for: digestion and constipation, said to act against digestive and colorectal cancers

Prunes
High in: fibre, beta-carotene, other anti-oxidants particularly anthocyanins
Good for: digestion, may act against digestive and colorectal cancers, can also help bowel disorders like diverticular disease

Pumpkin
High in: beta-carotene, vitamin C, potassium
Good for: prevention of arterial hardening, immunity, said to be anti-cancer, also helps curb the appetite

Radishes

High in: vitamin C, folic acid, magnesium, potassium

Good for: particular action against stomach cancer, energy boosting, may lower levels of homocysteine (a risk factor for heart disease)

Raisins

High in: iron, potassium, anti-oxidants and flavonoids including quercitin

Good for: energy levels, lowering blood pressure, may help prevent digestive cancers

Raspberries

High in: fibre, vitamin B2, vitamin B6, vitamin C, anti-oxidants – particularly ellagic acid

Good for: general digestive and all round health. Shows positive signs of helping prevent breast and stomach cancers

Seaweed

High in: iron, iodine, calcium, magnesium, phytoestrogens

Good for: bone health, hormone balancing, heart health, speeding the metabolism

Soya beans

High in: phytoestrogens

Good for: may help prevent breast cancer, regulates hormones, reduces menopausal symptoms

Spinach

High in: lutein, iron, folic acid, vitamin K

Good for: bone health, energy, eyesight – it is the number 1 preventor of macular degeneration

Squash

High in: beta-carotene, vitamin C, potassium

Good for: preventing cataracts, controls blood pressure, general health and immunity

Strawberries

High in: fibre, vitamin C, folic acid, calcium, anti-oxidants particularly ellagic acid

Good for: heart health, may help with breast and stomach cancers

Sweet potatoes

High in: beta-carotene, folic acid, copper, iron, calcium, vitamin C, vitamin E

Good for: heart health, energy levels, skin

Tomatoes

High in: vitamin C, calcium, iron, phosphorus, the carotenoid lycopene

Good for: heart health, said to be cancer fighting – particularly prostate, lung and cervical cancers

Watercress

High in: detoxifiers, anti-oxidants, chlorophyll

Good for: blood, energy levels, fighting effects of smoking

Watermelon

High in: vitamin C, beta-carotene, water, the carotenoid lycopene

Good for: fluid retention, may help fight lung and other cancers

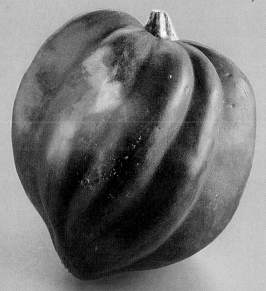

Index

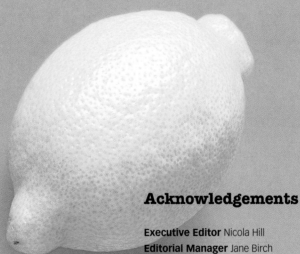

Acknowledgements

Executive Editor Nicola Hill
Editorial Manager Jane Birch
Executive Art Editor Geoff Fennell
Designer Brian Flynn
Production Controller Lucy Woodhead
Consultant Nutritionist Angie Jefferson
Photographer Stephen Conroy
Home Economist David Morgan
Stylist Angela Swaffield

All photographs © Octopus Publishing Group Ltd